Fortschritte der
Urologie und Nephrologie

Thomas C. Gasser

Antimicrobial Prophylaxis in Urology with special reference to the new Quinolones

Steinkopff Verlag Darmstadt

Thomas Gasser, M.D.
Urologic Clinics
Department of Surgery
University Hospital
(Kantonsspital)
4031 Basel
Switzerland

Die Deutsche Bibliothek – CIP-Einheitsaufnahme

Gasser, Thomas C.:
Antimicrobial prophylaxis in urology with special reference to the new quinolones / Thomas C. Gasser. – Darmstadt : Steinkopff, 1992
(Fortschritte der Urologie und Nephrologie)

ISBN-13:978-3-7985-0942-9 e-ISBN-13:978-3-642-85422-4
DOI: 10.1007/978-3-642-85422-4

Medical Editorial: Sabine Müller – English Editor: James C. Willis – Production: Heinz J. Schäfer

Typesetting: Typoservice, 6146 Alsbach

Printed on acid-free paper

Preface

This monograph gives an excellent review of the issue of antimicrobial prophylaxis in urology and the use of the new fluoroquinolones in urology. The development of the fluoroquinolones has had a profound effect in urology, specifically because of the unique pharmacokinetics of the fluoroquinolones with their two or more pK values, making concentration of these compounds possible in the prostate. Their wide spectra against infecting organisms causing infections in the urinary tract have also made them popular and almost ideal in the treatment of urinary tract infections.

This thesis summarizes in an concise way and brings up to date practically all our knowledge concerning the use of fluoroquinolones in urology. The chapter on antimicrobial prophylaxis covers our present knowledge completely, especially concerning the use of these drugs in antimicrobial prophylaxis in transurethral surgery.

September 1992

Paul O. Madsen
Madison, Wisconsin, USA

Contents

I. Introduction

1.1. Author's Publications Referred to in Text

This thesis is based on the following articles, referred to in the text by Roman numerals:

I. Gasser, T. C., Larsen, E. H., Dörflinger, T., Madsen, P. O.: The influence of various body fluids and pH on E. coli MIC of quinolone derivatives. In: Weidner W (ed). Therapy of Prostatitis. Zuckschwerdt Verlag, München, 50-53, 1986.

II. Gasser, T. C., Graversen, P. H., Larsen, E. H., Dörflinger, T.: Quinolone penetration into canine vaginal and urethral secretions. Scand. J. Urol. Nephrol. 104 (suppl): 101-105, 1987.

III. Gasser, T. C., Graversen, P. H., Madsen, P. O.: Fleroxacin (Ro 23-6240) distribution in canine prostatic tissue and fluids. Antimicrob. Agents Chemother. 31: 1010-1013, 1987.

IV. Gasser, T. C., Graversen, P. H., Larsen, E. H., Madsen, P. O.: Vergleichende Pharmakokinetik in der Prostata. In: Paul Ehrlich Gesellschaft (Naber KG, Adam D., Grobecker H., Hrsg.). Gyrase Hemmer II. Fortschritte der antimikrobiellen und antineoplastischen Chemotherapie. Futuramed Verlag, München, Band 6-10, 2027-2032, 1987.

V. Gasser, T. C., Ebert, S. C., Graversen, P. H., Madsen, P. O.: Ciprofloxacin pharmacokinetics in patients with normal and impaired renal function. Antimicrob. Agents Chemother. 31: 709-712, 1987.

VI. Gasser, T. C., Graversen, P. H., Madsen, P. O.: Treatment of complicated urinary tract infections with ciprofloxacin. Am. J. Med. 82 (suppl 4A): 278-279, 1987.

VII. Gasser, T. C., Madsen, P. O.: Antimicrobial prophylaxis in urology: Timing, dosing, and duration studies with special reference to high-risk conditions (unpublished).

1.2. Historical Background

Since the discovery of sulfa in the 1930's and penicillin in the 1940's, an enormous number of antimicrobials have been developed. Drugs, such as tetracyclines and cephalosporins, considerably improved the armory to fight bacterial infections. In the 1980's, one group of particularly interesting antimicrobials was introduced: the fluoroquinolones. They were developed from long known quinolones such as nalidixic acid, oxolinic acid, pipemidic acid, and cinoxacin. The fluorination of the molecule improved the antibacterial activity greatly (Hooper and Wolfson, 1991). As quinolones have been found to reach high tissue concentrations in genitourinary organs and have a very broad antibacterial spectrum, they have been successfully used to treat infections of the urinary tract (Nielsen and Madsen,

1989). For these reasons, quinolones appear to be suitable for prophylactic purposes in urology. However, as the benefit of antimicrobial prophylaxis in urology is highly disputed and different from any other area in medicine, a discussion of the role of quinolones with respect to antimicrobial prophylaxis seems warranted.

Antimicrobial agents have been used for prophylactic purposes for many years. But despite high expectations, early reports showed no benefit of antimicrobial prophylaxis (McKittrik and Wheelock, 1954). Some authors even found detrimental effects of prophylaxis, either owing to selection of resistant bacteria without reducing the number of infections (Sanchez-Ubeda et al., 1958), or to higher infection rates in the treatment group (National Research Council, 1964). It was only in 1961 when Burke's pioneer work provided the first scientific basis for rational use of prophylactic antimicrobials (Burke, 1961). He was able to show in a study of guinea pigs that infections of dermal lesions and experimental incisions could be prevented by antimicrobial agents. Most importantly, however, he found that antimicrobial agents had to be given before and no later than 3 hours after the incision. This finding led to change of the then accepted practice of administering the antimicrobial at termination of the operation.

1.3. Problems of Antimicrobial Prophylaxis in Urology

Since Burke's work, many clinical studies have proven the efficacy of antimicrobial prophylaxis in many surgical fields (Kaiser, 1986). The need for antimicrobial prophylaxis is undisputed for many operations and clinical conditions. Such conditions include operations with a high risk of infection, e.g., colonic surgery, or those in which infection causes high mortality (cardiac or vascular surgery), or serious morbidity (orthopedic surgery) (Guglielmo et al., 1983; Kaiser, 1986).

However, in urologic surgery, particularly transurethral surgery, much controversy remains as to the benefit of prophylactic administration of antimicrobials (Gasser et al., 1987; Grabe, 1987; Kaiser, 1986).

There may be various reasons for this controversy. First, Burke's work may only have limited applications in urology. Caution should be used when translating results of animal experiments to clinical situations. Burke's experiments were carried out in dermal lesions with Gram-positive organisms, whereas Gram-negative organisms are primarily encountered in clinical urology. While some authors have found no difference in infection rate between prophylactic and placebo groups (Ferrie and Scott, 1984; Qvist et al., 1984; Haverkorn, 1984), others have reported significant reductions in urinary tract infections and bacteremia in the treatment group (Prokocimer et al., 1986; Nielsen et al., 1981; Dörflinger and Madsen, 1984). Secondly, the efficacy of antimicrobial prophylaxis in urologic surgery is difficult to assess, as there are no clear definitions of postoperative infections such as wound infections or infection of a prosthesis. The definition of significant bacteriuria has been debated and appears to be 10^2 colony-forming units (CFU)/ml in catheterized patients, rather than the traditional level of 10^5 CFU/ml (Stark and Maki, 1984; see also chapter 2.1.1). Thirdly, many of the complications are minor and therefore, may be treated as they occur. Some urologists feel that it is safer to treat a urinary tract infection when it occurs according to the infecting organism than to administer antimicrobials to every patient.

Therefore, a review of the various aspects of antimicrobial prophylaxis in urologic surgery seems to be warranted.

II. General Considerations

2.1. Definitions

Infectious complications after urologic surgery usually follow a two-step pattern. The first step in urinary tract infection takes the form of a simple bladder infection. This may be symptomatic or asymptomatic, and the treatment is usually very effective. However, the infections secondary to this initial infection (in the form of bacteremia, septicemia, pyelonephritis, and wound infection) represent the real dangers to the patient. The two-step pattern is emphasized because patients with preoperatively infected urine have a much higher risk of acquiring a secondary infection. The incidence of infection is highly influenced by factors such as sex, age, type of instrumentation of the urinary tract, and general health condition. Because of wide inconsistencies in the literature, definitions and subsequent incidence of these infections are briefly discussed.

2.1.1. Bacteriuria and urinary tract infections

The term "bacteriuria" denotes the fact that any number of bacteria are found in the urine. Bacteriuria may be symptomatic or asymptomatic. If asymptomatic, the term "colonization" may be used. If symptoms are present, the term "urinary tract infection" (UTI) should be applied. The most often agreed upon level of significant bacteriuria is $> 10^5$ CFU/ml urine. This definition is based on studies by Kass, who found that women with $> 10^5$ CFU/ml in a clean voided urine specimen had a 80 % chance of having a true bladder infection (Kass, 1960). Colony counts of $< 10^5$ were considered contamination. However, newer studies indicate that the level of significant bacteriuria is considerably lower. One study of 122 catheterized patients found that a bacterial count of 10^3 CFU/ml was associated with pathological sequelae (Gordon et al., 1983). Another study reported that colony counts as low as 10^2 may represent an early stage of UTI (Stark and Maki, 1984). In this study, 96 % of patients with low-count bacteriuria developed UTI, usually within three days. On the other hand, when obtaining urine by suprapubic puncture, any bacteria detected are considered pathological. Unlike midstream urine (risk of contamination) and catheter urine (risk of introducing bacteria from the external meatus into the bladder), suprapubic puncture virtually assures no risk of false-positive results.

2.1.2. Bacteremia and septicemia

The terms "bacteremia", "septicemia", and "sepsis" are often used synonymously in the literature. Similar to bacteriuria, it is suggested that the presence of bacteria in the bloodstream be named "bacteremia", and symptomatic bacteremia should be named "septicemia.". However, any number of bacteria in the blood is considered pathological, as bacteremia is often transient (Biorn et al., 1950). Bacteremia following manipulation of the urinary tract occurs in up to 30 % of patients (Sullivan et al., 1973). Sullivan found that patients with preoperative indwelling catheter and UTI represented particular high-risk conditions with positive blood cultures in 50 % and 67 %, respectively. The secondary nature of bacteremia is illustrated by the finding that in 83 % of 221 bacteremic hospital-acquired infections, the same microorganisms were isolated from cultures of blood and urine (Bryan and Reynolds, 1984). Therefore, it is generally agreed that a UTI should be treated prior to any urologic operation (Kaiser, 1986).

2.1.3. Nosocomial infections

Nosocomial or hospital-acquired infections have been estimated in at least 5 % of patients admitted to hospitals in the U.S.A. (Haley et al., 1985b). More than 40 % of these infections are attributed to the urinary tract. An indwelling catheter in place for more than 3 days represents a major risk factor for nosocomial bacteremia (Trilla et al., 1991). Other major sites include surgical wounds (24 %), respiratory tract (10 %), blood (5 %), and other sites (19 %). Approximately 1 % of nosocomial UTI result in bacteremia, and 10 % of these are fatal (Stamm et al., 1977). In one study, the acquisition of a nosocomial UTI was associated with a threefold increase in hospital mortality (Platt et al., 1982). As illustrated in Table 1, about 75 % of nosocomial UTIs are due to Gram-negative bacteria. In a hospital setting, Escherichia coli accounts for approximately 50 % of these bacteriurias, followed by Proteus, Pseudomonas, Klebsiella, Enterobacter and Serratia. The remaining 25 % is largely due to Gram-positive organisms such as Streptococcus and Staphylococcus. Within the last decade, an increasing number of infections have been caused by more troublesome organisms such as Pseudomonas, Klebsiella, Serratia, Gram-positive cocci, and even Candida species (Krieger et al., 1983).

Table 1. Distribution of infecting organisms in 1,276 males undergoing transurethral resection of the prostate (TURP) at the Veterans Administration Hospital, Madison, WI (Nielsen et al., 1981)

Infecting Organism	Percentage With Infection
Escherichia coli	35.6
Proteus mirabilis	13.4
Streptococcus	12.6
Pseudomonas	10.8
Klebsiella	9.0
Staphylococcus	8.9
Indole-positive Proteus	3.8
Enterobacter	2.7
Citrobacter	1.6
Serratia	0.9
Providencia	0.7

2.1.4. Wound infections

Wound infections may be primary due to contamination at the site of incision or secondary through a remote infection such as UTI. The reported overall rate of wound infections in urologic patients has ranged from 2.3 % to 9.2 % (Cruse et al., 1980; Edwards, 1976). This is highly dependent on the type of surgery and degree of contamination of the wound. The National Research Council has created a classification of wounds and corresponding infection rates (National Research Council, 1964). According to this classification, Cruse studied more than 62,000 surgical wounds and found a "clean wound" infection rate of 1.5 % compared to a "dirty wound" rate of 40 % (Table 2) (Cruse et al., 1980).

While the benefit of antimicrobial prophylaxis in dirty wounds is undisputed, recent studies have also demonstrated reduced infection rates for clean operations like herniorrhaphy and certain types of breast surgery if antimicrobial prophylaxis is used (Platt et al., 1990). The importance of a remote infection has been stressed by Edwards who reported that the wound infection rate increased 2.7 to 5.3 times in patients with a secondary focus (Edwards, 1976). Among 1,865 patients with wound infections, he found a 61 % incidence of associated remote infections, the most frequent sites being the urinary tract (30 %), lower respiratory tract (25 %), gastrointestinal tract (11 %), and blood (9 %).

2.2. Pathophysiology of Infection

By administering antimicrobials prophylactically, prevention of possible or likely infection is attempted. This has to be clearly distinguished from therapy whereby infection has already occurred and is to be eradicated. Any operation causes a disruption of the natural barrier between a normally sterile tissue and the non sterile environment. In the case of an

Table 2. Classification of wounds (National Research Council, 1964; Cruse et al., 1980)

Classification	Definition	Wound Infection Rate (%)
Clean	No infection encountered, no break in aseptic technique, no hollow muscular organ opened	1.5
Clean contaminated	Hollow muscular organ opened, but minimal spillage of contents	7.7
Contaminated	Hollow muscular organ opened, gross spillage of contents or acute inflammation, major break in aseptic technique	15.2
Dirty	Pus encountered at operation or a perforated viscus found	40.0
Overall		4.7

open operation, the incision exposes the skin covered underlying tissue to the always contaminated air. In the case of endoscopic operations, the mucosa is traumatized and a direct communication between the cavity examined and the external environment is created (Larsen et al., 1986). Once the bacteria have gained access to the tissue, they may either multiply locally or enter the bloodstream and be carried to distant sites. Bacteria are defended by humoral and cellular mechanisms. However, if the number of invading organisms is exceedingly high or if the host's defense mechanisms are lowered for some reason, the bacteria may multiply and develop into a clinically evident infection. Therefore, the goal of antimicrobial prophylaxis is to reduce the number of bacteria in the body, thus supporting the natural defense mechanisms.

2.3. Specifics of Antimicrobial Agents to be Used in Prophylaxis

According to what was stated above, antimicrobials used for prophylactic purposes should possess the following properties:

- High efficacy against potentially invading bacteria
- Reach sufficient local tissue concentrations to inhibit bacterial growth
- Have pharmacokinetic properties to reach maximum concentration within a defined time frame
- Not being counteracted by the host environment, e.g., body fluids and pH
- Be effective against low, as well as high bacterial counts
- Not interfering with natural defense mechanisms due to local toxicity

Other properties such as lack of side effects, easy administration, and low cost must also be considered, although they are not prerequisites for successful prophylaxis.

2.4. Role of Quinolones

Since the discovery of the sulfonamides and penicillin, many new antimicrobial agents have been developed. Compared to the four antimicrobials tested by Burke (penicillin G, chloramphenicol, erythromycin, and achromycin), new agents have a broader antimicrobial spectrum, are less toxic, and easier to administer. One new groups of antimicrobials that are particularly interesting are the newer fluoroquinolones (Nielsen and Madsen, 1989). Their antimicrobial activity, pharmacokinetic properties, tissue concentration, and safety make the quinolones an attractive choice for prophylaxis in urology.

2.4.1. Antimicrobial activity

The antimicrobial activity, as well as pharmacokinetic properties of newer quinolones, have been outlined in detail elsewhere (Hooper and Wolfson, 1991). The basic structure of the fluoroquinolone antimicrobials is shown in Figure 1. The fluorine atom at position 6 is the hallmark of the fluoroquinolone and has considerably increased the antibacterial activity of the molecule, as compared to earlier groups of quinolones such as cinoxacin or

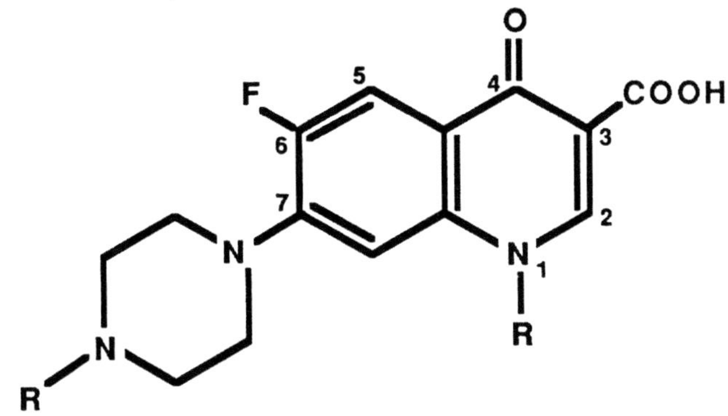

Fig. 1. Basic chemical structure of fluoroquinolones (R indicates side group).

nalidixic acid. The unique mode of action of quinolones is the binding and blocking of the bacterial DNA-gyrase enzyme. This prevents the supercoiling of the DNA molecule, which is necessary for the bacterium to function. The gyrase in human cells is different and, therefore, not inhibited by the quinolones.

The MIC of various quinolones against selected bacteria is listed in Table 3. In general, quinolones are active against Gram-positive and Gram-negative bacteria, including several Pseudomonas strains and beta-lactam bacteria. The antibacterial spectrum includes most of the uropathogens. Gram-positive cocci, Chlamydia trachomatis, and Ureaplasma urealyticum are usually less sensitive, and anaerobic bacteria are resistant to quinolones. Despite wide use, development of resistance appears to be low (Kresken and Wiedemann, 1988). The influence of various factors (pH, body fluid, inoculum size) on quinolone MIC is discussed in section 3.2.

2.4.2. Pharmacokinetic properties

Some fluoroquinolones can be administered both orally and intravenously (Höffken et al., 1985). The absolute oral bioavailability is rapid and exceeds 50 %. It is greatest in ofloxacin and pefloxacin (> 95 %). The absorption is delayed by food or antacids (Ledergerber et al., 1985; Preheim et al, 1986). Quinolones reach very high concentrations in serum, e.g., up to 4.2 μg/ml for ciprofloxacin, and urine (up to 500 μg/ml). They are well tolerated after sequential dose increases (Tartaglione et al., 1986). The distribution volume exceeds 1 L/kg, indicating excellent tissue penetration (Weidekamm et al., 1987). The terminal half-life of most quinolones has been calculated to be between 3 and 5 hours, except for fleroxacin and pefloxacin which have half-lives of 11.2 and 10.5 hours, respectively (Hooper and Wolfson, 1991; Weidekamm et al., 1987).

Elimination of quinolones is both renal and nonrenal. In an open, randomized, crossover study of 32 men with impaired renal function, we found that reducing the dose of ciprofloxacin was necessary only if creatinine clearance was below 50 ml/min (V). However, in patients with severely impaired renal function, ciprofloxacin was still excreted renally and reached concentrations several times higher than the MIC for most urinary pathogens, suggesting clinical efficacy in this group of patients.

2.4.3. Side effects

Quinolones are usually well tolerated. Side effects occur in approximately 5 %. Gastrointestinal and central nervous system side effects prevail, but are usually mild (Nielsen and Madsen, 1989). Allergic reactions have been infrequently reported. Studies have shown cartilage damage in young animals given quinolones. Children, pregnant, and breastfeeding women should therefore not be treated with fluoroquinolones. Many fluoroquinolones, especially enoxacin, ciprofloxacin, and pefloxacin, interfere with the hepatic metabolism of theophylline by lowering its clearance, leading to possible overdose (Hooper and Wolfson, 1991). Crystalluria has also been reported but is usually not of clinical relevance.

Table 3. Activity of fluoroquinolones in vitro against common uropathogens (µg/ml) . [a] (Adapted from Hooper and Wolfson, 1991; Nielsen and Madsen, 1989)

	NORFLOX	CIPRO	OFLOX	ENOX	PEFLOX	FLEROX	LOMEFLOX
Escherichia coli	0.12	0.03	0.12	0.40	0.25	1.00	0.25
Proteus mirabilis	0.10	<0.12	0.20	0.80	0.50	0.50	–
Streptococcus pyogenes	6.30	2.00	3.10	12.00	–	16.00	8.00
Pseudomonas aeruginosa	2.00	0.50	2.00	4.00	2.00	2.00	4.00
Klebsiella pneumoniae	1.60	<0.12	0.20	3.10	2.00	2.00	–
Staphylococcus aureus	6.30	1.00	0.40	3.10	0.50	1.00	2.00
Coagulase-negative Staphylococcus	3.10	0.25	0.80	6.30	0.50	1.00	1.00
Enterobacter	0.40	<0.12	1.00	0.40	–	2.00	–
Serratia marcescens	3.10	1.00	1.60	6.30	1.00	12.00	2.00
Bacteroides fragilis	>128	8.00	8.00	32.00	16.00	32.00	32.00
Neisseria gonorrhea	0.06	0.01	0.06	0.25	–	0.20	0.12
Chlamydia trachomatis	25.00	1.60	0.80	6.30	–	3.10	3.20

[a]MIC 90 (concentration of drug inhibiting 90 % of strains tested).
NORFLOX = Norfloxacin, CIPRO = Ciprofloxacin, OFLOX = Ofloxacin, PEFLOX = Pefloxacin, FLEROX = Fleroxacin, LOMEFLOX = Lomefloxacin

2.4.4. Uncomplicated urinary tract infection

Treatment of uncomplicated UTI is simple and highly effective. Single-dose treatment appears to be as effective as treatment over several days (Fang et al., 1978). Newer quinolones have shown cure rates comparable to or better than trimethoprim sulfamethoxazole in the treatment of acute cystitis. In one study, the overall bacterial cure rate for single use of norfloxacin, ciprofloxacin, ofloxacin, fleroxacin, and pefloxacin was 83 % (Andriole, 1991). With a three-dose regimen, slightly better cure rates were achieved. Conversely, in a study of 209 patients with uncomplicated UTI, a ten-day treatment with norfloxacin did not produce higher cure rates as compared to a three-day regimen (Stein et al., 1987).

The emergence of resistant bacteria appears to be of minor importance with quinolones. In a study of 40 women with uncomplicated UTI who were treated for 10 days, norfloxacin was as effective and safe as trimethoprim (Schaeffer and Sisney, 1985). However, no resistant bacteria were observed in the norfloxacin treated group as compared to 11 % in the trimethoprim treated group.

Nevertheless, because of the excellent cure rates of conventional drugs such as trimethoprim and amoxicillin, fluoroquinolones should be restricted to difficult-to-treat UTI.

The role of newer quinolones in the prophylaxis of recurrent UTI has yet to be determined. Long-term, low-dose norfloxacin has increased the interval between symptomatic attacks by 26 % over a 12-month period (Brumfitt et al., 1989). No resistance has emerged during the 12 months of continuous therapy; however, nitrofurantoin was as effective as norfloxacin, yet had no effect on intestinal flora.

2.4.5. Complicated urinary tract infection

Complicated UTI is defined as an infection in the presence of a structural or functional abnormality of the urinary tract. Generally, the fluoroquinolones achieve cure rates equal or higher than conventional drugs (Naber, 1989). In a study of 43 women, no significant difference in cure rates was found between norfloxacin (400 mg bid) and trimethoprim-sulfamethoxasole (160 – 800 mg bid) (95 % and 90 %, respectively [Haase et al., 1984]). In another study, ofloxacin was equally effective as trimethoprim-sulfamethoxazole but clearly superior to carbenicillin (Cox, 1989). In a study of 45 women with complicated UTI, cure rates of ciprofloxacin were significantly higher than of trimethoprim-sulfamethoxazole (82 % vs 52 %, respectively, [Allais et al., 1988]).

We performed a study on 161 patients with complicated UTI (VI). The safety and efficacy of a three-dose regimen of ciprofloxacin (250, 500, and 750 mg orally every 12 hours for 7 days) were compared in a prospective, controlled, randomized, double-blind study. Cure rates 7 days after treatment were approximately 85 % with no differences among groups, suggesting that 250 mg of ciprofloxacin twice daily is sufficient for the treatment of UTI.

Treatment results with ofloxacin and enoxacin are generally not different from those using ciprofloxacin or norfloxacin (Cox, 1989; Naber, 1989).

2.4.6. Bacterial prostatitis

Prostatitis is a disease often misdiagnosed and therefore, mistreated. Drach et al. (1978) introduced a classification of prostatitis based on objective evidence of the microscopic examination of urine and prostatic secretion (Meares and Stamey, 1968). Voided urine and prostatic secretions are collected and cultured in segmented specimens: the first 10 ml voided (voided bladder 1 [VB1]); the midstream sample (VB2); the expressed prostatic secretion (EPS) obtained by prostatic massage; and the first 10 ml voided immediately after prostatic message (VB3). The diagnosis of prostatic infection is confirmed when the quantitative bacterial colony count of the prostatic specimens (EPS and VB3) significantly exceeds those of urethral (VB1) and bladder (VB2) specimens. According to the classification suggested by Drach et al., only acute and chronic bacterial prostatitis are caused by bacterial infection of the prostate. The etiology of nonbacterial prostatitis and prostatodynia is not clear. Nonbacterial prostatitis clearly shows signs of inflammation in the absence of bacteria. Infecting agents such as Chlamydia trachomatis (Doble et al., 1989) and Ureaplasma urealyticum (Berger et al., 1989) have been suggested, but never proven. Prostatodynia appears to be a urodynamic problem rather than an infection of the prostate (Barbalias et al., 1983).

The treatment of acute bacterial prostatitis usually poses no particular problems. As it is most often caused by Gram-negative enterobacteria such as Escherichia coli, Proteus mirabilis, Klebsiella pneumoniae, and Pseudomonas aeruginosa, quinolones are expected to be highly effective. Treatment should be instituted immediately and continued for 3–4 weeks to prevent prostatic abscess and chronic bacterial prostatitis. Conversely, chronic bacterial prostatitis is difficult to treat. Best cure rates range from 32 % to 71 % with trimethoprim (Meares, 1980). This has been explained by poor drug penetration into the prostate (Stamey et al., 1970; see also section 4.1). Newer quinolones concentrate in the prostate, making them ideal drugs for the treatment of chronic bacterial prostatitis (IV). Ofloxacin has been shown to be superior to carbenicillin (the only antimicrobial approved by the American Food and Drug Administration for this indication until a few years ago) (Cox, 1989). Ciprofloxacin has also been used successfully (Weidner, 1987). Bacterial prostatitis is a rare disease at present, but is expected to increase as more patients acquire the AIDS syndrome (Leport et al., 1989). Therefore, the importance of quinolones in the treatment of this disease will also increase.

2.5. Cost-Benefit Analysis of Antimicrobial Prophylaxis

Worldwide, antimicrobial agents are increasingly used and often misused. For example, one study reported that only 38 % of patients receiving antimicrobials had recorded evidence of infection (Scheckler and Bennett, 1970). Beside the morbidity and discomfort to the patient, cost-benefit analysis is an increasingly important factor to be considered. In 1990, over 15 billion U.S. dollars were spent worldwide on antimicrobial agents alone (Kunin et al., 1990). Therefore, indiscriminate use of antimicrobials raises the costs of an already strained health care system. On the other hand, physicians are increasingly faced with lawsuits for malpractice, prompting them to be more cautious and overprescribe antimicrobials. This may be reflected by the fact that the rate of antimicrobial agent misuse is higher in surgical services than in medical services (Weiner et al., 1980).

Urologic surgery is performed with increasing frequency, with transurethral prostatectomy being the most common procedure (Rutkow, 1982). Approximately 400,000 transurethral resections of the prostate (TURP) are performed each year in the U.S. alone, making it the tenth most frequent of all operations (Rutkow, 1986).

Assuming that 30 % of patients who undergo TURP acquire infections, approximately 120,000 UTI can be attributed to this kind of surgery annually (Larsen et al., 1986). In 1985, one nosocomial UTI was estimated to prolong a hospital stay by 2.5 days at an extra cost of $ 355 (Rutledge and McDonald, 1985; Haley et al., 1981b). Therefore, the additional costs of nosocomial UTI in connection with TURP may exceed 43 million dollars annually in the U.S. Similar data for Switzerland are not available. Assuming a similar rate of surgery as in other western countries, approximately 10,000 TURP are performed in Switzerland, resulting in up to 3,000 nosocomial UTI. If the daily hospital cost in Switzerland is 300 Swiss francs/day ($ 200 in U.S.), extra costs may exceed 2.3 million Swiss francs annually. On the other hand, if every patient is given a single injection of a newer cephalosporin (e.g., cefotaxime, $ 25/g), the approximate prophylaxis cost is 12 million dollars in the U.S. and 160,000 francs in Switzerland. If cheaper drugs such as first-generation cephalosporins are administered (e.g., cefazolin), costs may be reduced to one-tenth of this figure. The cost of quinolones compares favorably with that of cephalosporins, e.g., a single treatment of 750 mg ciprofloxacin costs approximately $ 3.50 (Hooper and Wolfson, 1991). Therefore, with successful prophylaxis, huge amounts of money could be saved. Admittedly, such calculations are theoretical and do not take into account individual factors such as patient morbidity, type of surgery, surgeon proficiency, etc. Moreover, complete prevention of infectious complications is not possible with antimicrobial prophylaxis. But even a partial reduction in infection would result in considerable savings of precious health care funds.

III. In Vitro Studies

3.1. Minimal Inhibitory Concentrations (MIC)

The most frequent pathogens encountered in urologic surgery are Gram-negative bacteria (Table 1). In a hospital setting, E. coli is still the predominant pathogen, but bacteria that are difficult to treat such as Proteus mirabilis and Pseudomonas aeruginosa are found with increasing frequency. Third-generation cephalosporins have been widely used for prophylaxis as they have a favorable antimicrobial action and low toxicity (McEniry and Gorbach, 1987). The MIC against most uropathogens is well below 1 mg/L for most third-generation cephalosporins. Likewise, quinolones have a very broad antimicrobial spectrum against most uropathogens and some are active against Pseudomonas aeruginosa, Staphylococcus aureus, Mycoplasma and Chlamydia trachomatis (Hooper and Wolfson, 1991; Nielsen and Madsen, 1989). Moreover, the quinolone MIC against many of these bacteria is very low (see Table 3 and section 2.4.1).

3.2. Influence of Various Factors on MIC (I)

The MIC is usually determined under standardized in vitro conditions with an inoculum size of 10^5 CFU in a medium with a pH of 7.2. However, in the living organism the number of bacteria and the pH may be different, and there may be interaction between body fluid and antimicrobial agents.

The materials and methods, as well as the results of a study addressing these questions are detailed in paper I. In brief, the MIC of various quinolones was only slightly affected by either very high or very low numbers of bacteria (no inoculum effect). Conversely, an increase of the inoculum from 10^6 to 10^9 caused a 19-fold increase in trimethoprim MIC. While the MIC for most quinolones studied was higher in canine prostatic fluid and tissue, and in human urine, such an increase could not be demonstrated in human prostatic tissue. Decreases in MIC ranging between 11- and 42-fold for all the quinolones studied occurred between pH 5.7 and 7.0. However, further increases in pH only affected the MIC slightly for most quinolones, except amifloxacin. This relatively stable antimicrobial activity of quinolones explains why these drugs are highly active in humans and therefore, are also expected to be beneficial for prophylactic purposes. The increase in MIC in human urine is of no clinical importance, as very high urine concentrations are achieved with all quinolones (Hooper and Wolfson, 1991).

IV. Animal Studies

4.1. Drug Penetration into Various Tissues (II, III, IV)

In order to achieve antibacterial activity, an antimicrobial agent must reach tissue concentrations above the MIC of that drug against the bacteria. Concentrations of various quinolones in prostatic tissue, prostatic fluid, and vaginal and urethral secretions were examined in a canine model (II, III, IV). Briefly, the drug was given intravenously to achieve steady-state conditions. At various intervals, samples of vaginal, urethral, and prostatic secretions were taken. At the end of the study, the animals were sacrificed. The

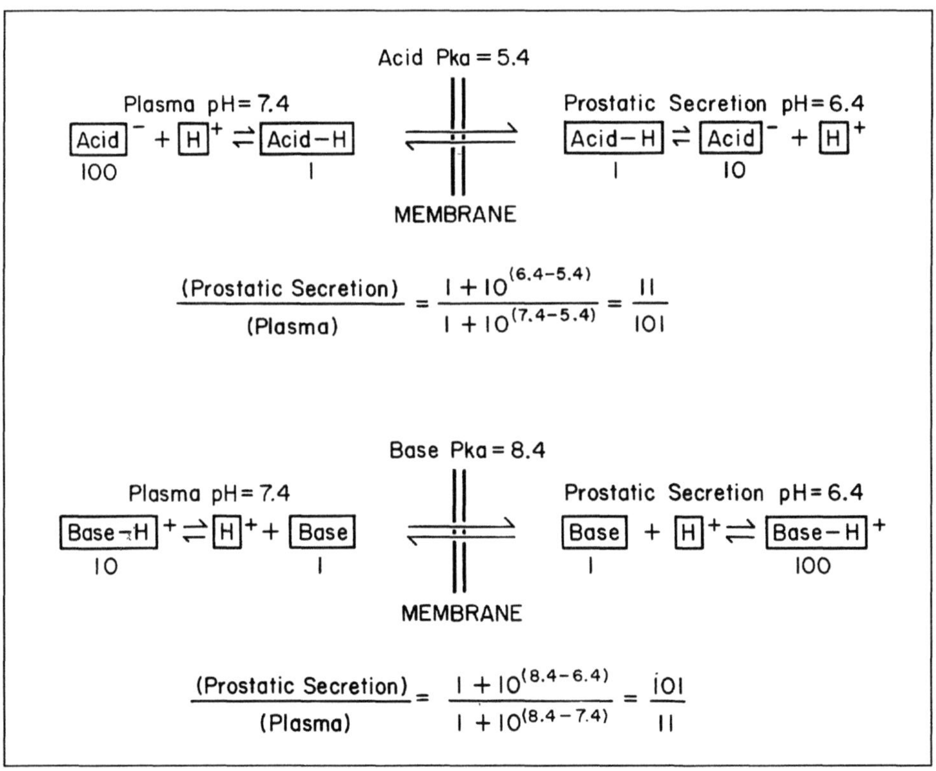

Fig. 2. Illustration of non-ionic diffusion of an antibacterial acid (pK_a 5.4) and an antibacterial base (pK_a 8.4) into dog prostatic fluid. (adapted from Stamey et al., 1970)

organs were removed and homogenized, and drug concentrations were determined by bioassay. These studies demonstrated that all of the quinolones reached very high tissue concentrations, sometimes several times higher than the plasma concentration.

It is not known how many times above the MIC the tissue concentration must be to be effective. It seems logical that the higher the concentration, the better. The term “inhibitory quotient“ or “therapeutic index“ has been suggested to express this ratio: drug concentration divided by MIC 90 (Ellner and Neu, 1981). The new quinolones achieve very high therapeutic indices, e.g., 340 for ciprofloxacin in the prostate (III). This high number demonstrates the excellent combination of high tissue concentration and low MIC. The findings in these animal studies have been confirmed in humans. Quinolones reach very high concentrations in most tissues (Gerding and Hitt, 1989), particularly in the prostate and prostatic tissue (Boerema et al., 1985).

Drug penetration into the prostate gland is thought to be governed by the principles determining drug passage across biological lipid-containing membranes in general. In the absence of secretory or active transport mechanisms, the drug penetration is presumably

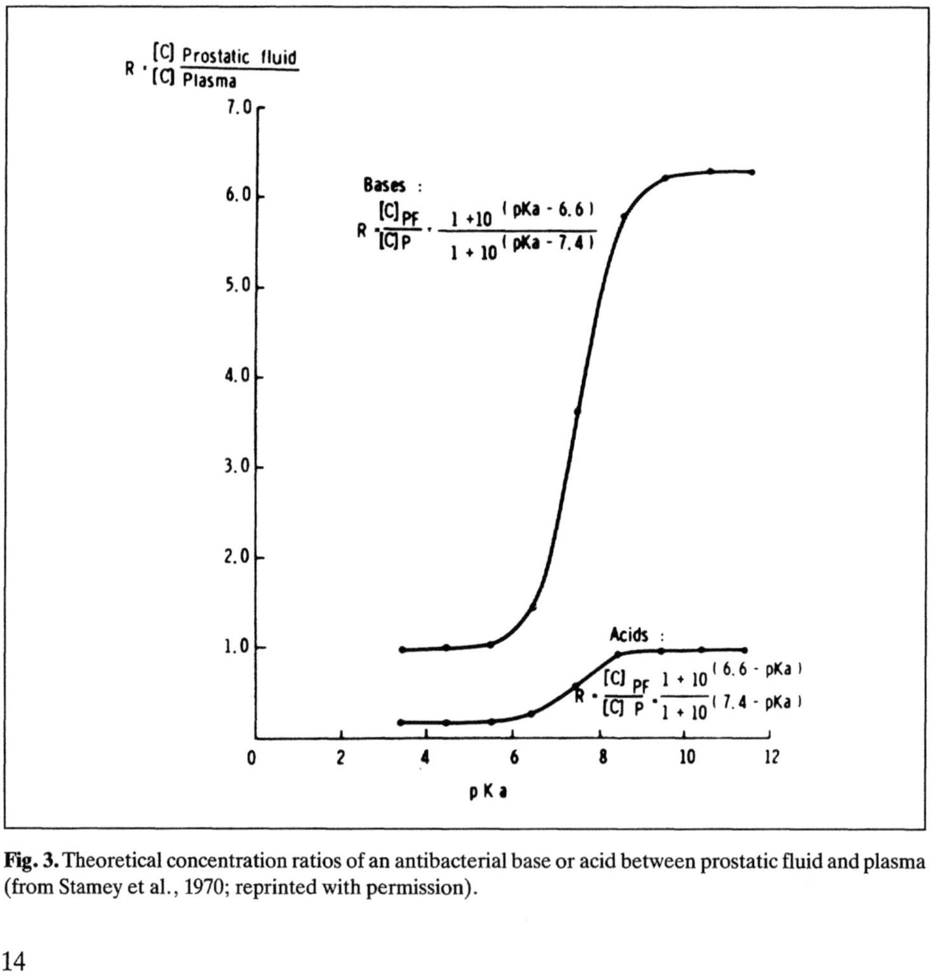

Fig. 3. Theoretical concentration ratios of an antibacterial base or acid between prostatic fluid and plasma (from Stamey et al., 1970; reprinted with permission).

passive, consisting of diffusion and concentration. Drug characteristics that determine simple diffusion and concentration are lipid solubility, degree of ionization, degree of protein binding, and the size and shape of the molecule. In addition, the presence of a pH gradient across a biological membrane induces the phenomenon of ion trapping. In the dog prostate, there is a pH gradient across the prostatic epithelium, the pH of plasma being 7.4 and of the prostatic secretion being 6.4 (Figure 2). In a stable system, the uncharged fraction of a lipid soluble drug will equilibrate on the two sides of the membrane but the charged fraction will vary, depending on the pH, the higher drug concentration being on the side of the higher degree of ionization.

The Henderson-Hasselbalch equation determines the theoretical drug concentration ratio across a biological membrane at equilibrium. In the Henderson-Hasselbalch equation ($pH = pK_a + \log [A^-]/[AH]$), pH relates to the medium, pK_a is the ionization constant, $[A^-]$ and $[AH]$ are the concentrations of ionized and non-ionized fractions of the drug, respectively (Madsen et al., 1986).

Figure 3 illustrates the situation for an acid with pK_a of 5.4 and a base with pK_a of 8.4. The higher the pK_a is for an acid, the higher the drug concentration will be in the prostatic secretion, but it will never exceed the plasma concentration. Weak bases, however, may concentrate (exceed plasma concentrations) in the prostatic secretion and the higher the pK_a, the higher the drug concentration will be.

The newer quinolones are amphoteric or zwitterionic drugs. Figure 4 shows the ionization curves of an acid (cinoxacin), a base (trimethoprim), and the amphoteric quinolones (ciprofloxacin and temafloxacin). The curves were calculated using the Henderson-Has-

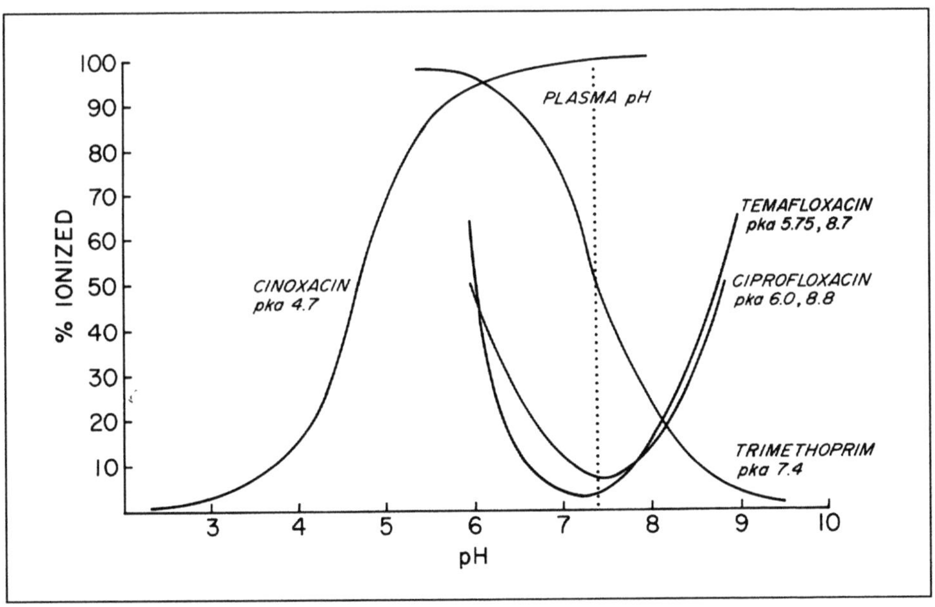

Fig. 4. Theoretical concentration curves for an acid (cinoxacin), a base (trimethoprim) and amphoteric substances (ciprofloxacin, temafloxacin), calculated using the Henderson-Hasselbalch equation [adapted from IV].

selbalch equation. Most amphoteric quinolones have two ionization groups, one positively charged and one negatively charged. At the isoelectric point, representing the average of the two pK_a values, the ionization is at a minimum. Since the best drug diffusion into the prostate occurs at the site lowest in degree of ionization, drugs with an isoelectric point close to plasma pH will diffuse well into the prostate. Conversely, amphoteric drugs with an isoelectric point different from the pH of plasma will diffuse poorly into the prostate.

4.2. Timing, Dosing, and Duration Studies (VII)

Since Burke's animal studies 30 years ago, many clinical studies have demonstrated the benefits of some kind of antimicrobial prophylaxis in various settings (Burke, 1961; Kaiser, 1986). Despite the enormous amount of new antimicrobial agents, few experimental studies addressing such basic issues as timing, dosing, and duration of antimicrobial prophylaxis have been published. In 1980, one animal study on prophylaxis in a fulgurated bladder found that appropriate timing varied with the infecting organism (Bagley et al., 1980). This study also demonstrated that persistent bacteriuria depends on the size of the bacterial inoculum and that a single dose of an antimicrobial possibly prevents infection. Another study on rats could not confirm Burke's "decisive period" (Burke, 1961), as prophylaxis was effective up to 6 hours after bacterial challenge (Nielsen and Madsen, 1982). Also in this study, the infecting organism and infected organs appeared to be of great importance. Single-dose antimicrobial prophylaxis considerably lowered the infecting rate in kidney and epididymis, and eliminated the infection completely in the prostate.

We performed a guinea pig study to investigate the importance of timing, dosing, and duration of antimicrobial prophylaxis (VII). To simulate high-risk conditions in some animals, we subcutaneously implanted a plastic chamber in the flank to serve as a foreign body 4 weeks before experiments were conducted. After cauterizing the prostate, bacteremia was induced by an intravenously administered solution of E. coli containing 2.7 x 10^5 CFU/ml. The animals were sacrificed after 24 hours, and organs were removed under sterile conditions and examined for bacteria.

In the timing study, ciprofloxacin was administered 15 min before, during, and 15 min and 3 hours after bacteremia induction. In the dosing study, ciprofloxacin was given at full dose (5.7 mg/kg), one-fourth of the dose, and one-eighth of the dose. To investigate duration, a triple-dose ciprofloxacin regimen was compared to a single dose.

This study confirmed the efficacy of prophylactic administration of a newer quinolone. However, it appeared that the decisive period for efficacy is even shorter than 3 hours. A single dose was as effective as multiple doses. One-fourth of the recommended dose was equally effective, but one-eighth was not. The infection of the foreign body could reliably be prevented with single dose antimicrobials.

In summary, this study confirmed the efficacy of antimicrobial prophylaxis for newer quinolones and the current trend to apply antimicrobial prophylaxis for a limited time only. The antimicrobials should be given before the bacterial challenge. This finding recently has been confirmed in a large clinical setting (Classen et al., 1992).

4.3. Bladder Irrigation Studies

It is known that bacterial adhesion to the bladder mucosa is the first step to infection (Svanborg Edén et al., 1976).

During a transurethral operation, a non-ionic, and therefore nonconductive, irrigation fluid is used. Various commercial solutions are available. But while many studies address the question of prophylactic antimicrobials little is known as to the importance of irrigation solutions for the development of postoperative urinary tract infection. Iversen and Madsen (1982) had found that high intravesical pressure irrigation led to higher bacterial adherence while change of temperature did not.

The influence of some of the most common irrigation fluids on bacterial adherence to the bladder mucosa has been studied in a in vitro and a guinea pig model (Gasser and Madsen, 1992, submitted for publication). The irrigation solutions studied were glycine 1.5 %, glycine 1.5 % and ethanol 1 %, glycerol 3 %, mannose 6 %, sorbitol 2.7 % and mannitol 0.54 %. Povidone-iodine and normal saline were used as controls.

The in vitro studies showed that while all irrigation fluids had some antibacterial activity it was most pronounced for mannose 6 % where after 120 minutes only 48 % of the original inoculum of 3.4×10^5 CFU was present. This was most likely because mannose was the only solution effectively blocking the type I pili of the Escherichia coli strain used. Type I pili are the most widely found type of bacterial adhesins.

In the guinea pig study two different strains of E. coli were tested: one with type I pili and one without. After electrocautery of one bladder side the bladder was incoculated with 10^8 CFU E. coli for 30 minutes. Then the bladder was irrigated with various solutions. It was found that E. coli with type I pili adhered clearly stronger to the bladder urothelium than E. coli without that adhesin. Moreover, it was found that the type I containing E. coli particularly adhered to urothelium injured by electocautery. This suggests that the more virulent bacteria also adhere stronger to the injured site of the bladder. No statistically significant difference was found among the irrigation solutions. Considering the in vivo results it appears, however, that mannose 6 % may be superior to the other investigated solutions in preventing postoperative urinary tract infection, possibly because of its anti-adherence effect.

V. Human Studies and Review of the Literature

Studies of antimicrobial prophylaxis in urologic surgery are numerous and will be discussed according to the various kinds of surgery employed. Prophylactic studies using quinolones are relatively sparse, but are being published with increasing frequency. Childs (1983) suggested that urologic procedures should be classified according to designations of wound infection as determined by the National Research Council (1964). Table 4 gives an overview of suggested classifications of urologic procedures and corresponding recommendations for prophylaxis. Only in clean operations is antimicrobial prophylaxis usually not necessary. In clean-contaminated procedures and contaminated procedures, single-

Table 4. Recommendations for antimicrobial prophylaxis in urologic surgery.

Operative Wound Classification	Corresponding Urologic Procedure	Recommendation[a]
Clean	– Operation of external genitalia – Simple nephrectomy – Catheterization/urethral dilatation – Cystoscopy/simple retrograde pyelography – Transperineal prostate biopsy – Laparoscopic surgery – ESWL	No prophylaxis
Clean-contaminated	– Pyeloplasty – TURP/TURB/Internal Urethrotomy – Ureterorenoscopy – Percutaneous nephrolitholapaxy – Transrectal prostate biopsy – Partial cystectomy	Single-dose prophylaxis
Contaminated	– Open prostatectomy/Radical prostatectomy – Cystectomy and urinary diversion with proper bowel preparation – Kidney transplantation – Insertion of prosthesis or foreign body – Stone surgery	Short-time prophylaxis (3-5 days)
Dirty	– Any procedure following acute trauma – TURP/TURB in the presence of bacteriuria – Urinary diversion in the absence of adequate bowel preparation	Prophylaxis followed by treatment regimen

[a] Patients with defective or artificial heart valves should be treated according to guidelines (Malinverni et al., 1984; Simmons et al., 1982) for the prevention of subacute endocarditis.

dose and short-time (3–5 days) prophylaxis, respectively, should suffice. Dirty wounds require antimicrobial prophylaxis, followed by prolonged therapeutic antimicrobial administration.

5.1. Catheterization and Urethral Dilatation

Urinary catheters are used for various reasons, from relieving urinary retention to monitoring urinary output in a critically ill patient, to control of bleeding after TURP. The risk of bacteriuria after a single catheterization is 2 % in an outpatient setting (Walter and Vejlsgaard, 1978). This rate increases to 20 % for inpatients (Garibaldi et al., 1974; Thiel and Spühler, 1965). Nineteen percent of patients on the urology ward are treated with indwelling catheters (Wenzel et al., 1976). Eighty percent of nosocomial UTI are attributed to indwelling catheters (Stamm et al., 1977). The risk of infection increases with the duration of the catheterization. The cumulative risk of infection has been estimated to exceed 5 % per day, with all patients becoming infected after approximately 10 days (Figure 5; Fowler, 1983).

In a catheterized patient, bacteria may gain access to the bladder by the intra- or extraluminal pathway. Entrance via the intraluminal pathway was dramatically reduced by the introduction of a closed drainage system, reducing the infection rate from 95 % to

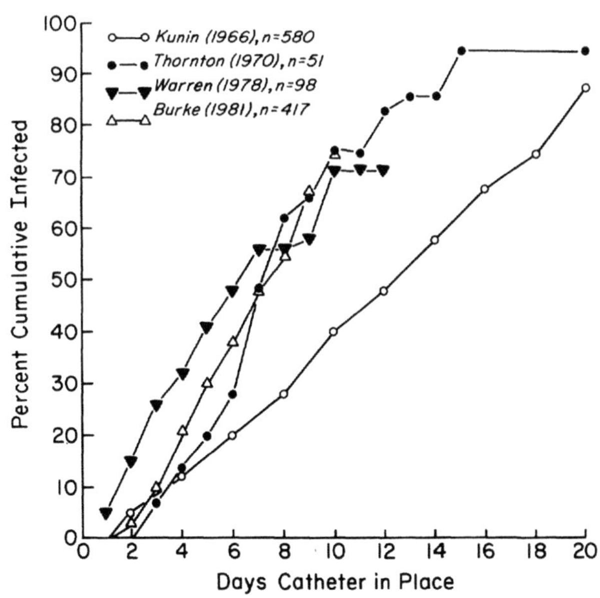

Fig. 5. Cumulative percentage of catheterized patients acquiring urinary tract infection.

23 % (Kunin and McCormack, 1966). The existence of the extraluminal pathway was demonstrated by Kass who, after inoculating the urethral meatus with Serratia marcescens, was able to isolate the same organism in the urine two days later (Kass and Schneidermann, 1957). Ascending bacteria move along the catheter by building a biofilm at a speed of approximately 1 cm/hr (Nickel et al., 1992). The bacteria ascending the periurethral mucous sheath originate from meatal colonization and the perineum (Garibaldi et al., 1980; Brehmer and Madsen, 1972). Also, the anterior urethra is often a source of bacteria leading to UTI after instrumentation (Walker et al., 1986). Various measures to reduce the intra- and extraluminal pathways have been described. Indications for placing a catheter should be strict, and the catheter should be indwelling for the shortest possible time. The closed drainage system should be applied, and disconnection of the catheter bag junction should be avoided, as this is associated with high risk of infection (Kunin and McCormack, 1966; Warren et al., 1978). Trials in which disinfectant agents were placed in the drainage bag produced conflicting results, but may reduce UTI (Holliman et al., 1987; Maizels and Schaeffer, 1980; Thompson et al., 1984). Brehmer and Madsen (1972) found contamination of the drainage bag was of minor importance. On the other hand, they found a reduced infection rate in patients who had daily antiseptic sitz baths and applied an antibiotic spray to the perineum and external genitalia. Conversely, other authors found no benefit of daily meatal care (Burke et al., 1981; Classen et al., 1991). The use of an antiseptic lubricating gel may be effective in preventing UTI following catheterization (Cohen, 1985).

Systemic antimicrobial agents reduce the frequency of bacteriuria, but the protection only lasts for the first four days of catheterization (Garibaldi et al., 1974). However, if infection has occurred, removal of the catheter alone is not sufficient, and administration of antimicrobials is necessary to clear the infection (Gordon et al., 1983). One must consider that long-term antimicrobial administration increases the risk of development of bacterial resistance (Mountokalakis et al., 1985). Also, it has been shown that the short-term use of an indwelling catheter after extensive surgery reduces the incidence of urinary retention and bladder over-distension, without increasing the rate of UTI (Michelson et al., 1988). To reduce infection, an alternate urinary drainage system should be considered. Clean intermittent self-catheterization has been used successfully in patients with voiding dysfunction, resulting in reduced infection rate as compared to patients with indwelling catheters (Lapides et al., 1974). Use of suprapubic catheterization can reduce UTI considerably (Shapiro et al., 1982). No data are available on the infection risk of urethral dilatation to treat urethral stricture. It is assumed that the risk of UTI matches that of simple catheterization. If dilatation has been difficult and traumatizing, antimicrobial prophylaxis may be necessary. Therefore, antimicrobial prophylaxis is only needed for high-risk patients (those with defective or artificial heart valves).

5.2. Endourologic Procedures

5.2.1. Cystoscopy

Theoretically, a gentle diagnostic cystoscopy with a small (17 French) endoscope should carry no higher infection rate than a single catheterization. However, since Barrington and Wright (1930) found that transient bacteremia is very common after urethral manipulation, routine antimicrobial prophylaxis has been instituted in many centers. A 10 % – 16 %

incidence of chills or rigors was reported in patients undergoing ambulatory cystoscopy, but no blood cultures were obtained (Hart et al., 1980; Reilly et al., 1981). The 10 % incidence of chills in the group undergoing prophylaxis suggested endotoxin release rather than true bacteremia. One study, however, demonstrated a reduction in UTI of 45 % to 2 % following endoscopy when sulfa-trimethoprim was administered as compared to placebo (Korbel and Maher, 1976). However, newer prospective randomized trials showed an overall infection rate of 2 % with no differences between the treated and control groups (Manson, 1988). The latter finding is in accordance with everyday clinical practice. Hence, antimicrobial prophylaxis is not recommended for patients with sterile urine who undergo cystoscopy. In case of UTI, pathogen-specific antimicrobial therapy should be instituted and cystoscopy should be delayed until the infection has cleared.

5.2.2. Internal urethrotomy

Literature that specifically addresses urethrotomy is sparse. One study of 23 patients showed a possible advantage of oral ciprofloxacin over no prophylaxis (Murdoch and Badenoch, 1987). As the risk and mechanism of infection appear to be similar to those in other kinds of transurethral surgery, these problems will be discussed in detail in the following sections.

5.2.3. Transurethral resection of the prostate (TURP)

TURP is the most frequent urologic procedure performed in the U.S. (Rutkow, 1986). Therefore, it is the most widely investigated regarding the benefit of antimicrobial prophylaxis. Infectious complications (UTI and septicemia) were the most common in a study of 1,000 patients who underwent TURP (Paquin et al., 1988).

Possible sources of infection are shown in figure 6 and include the inevitable lens-eye contact, the urethra with its wide variety of bacteria (Garibaldi et al., 1974), the prostate (Gorelick et al., 1988), and contaminated irrigation fluids (Morris et al., 1976).

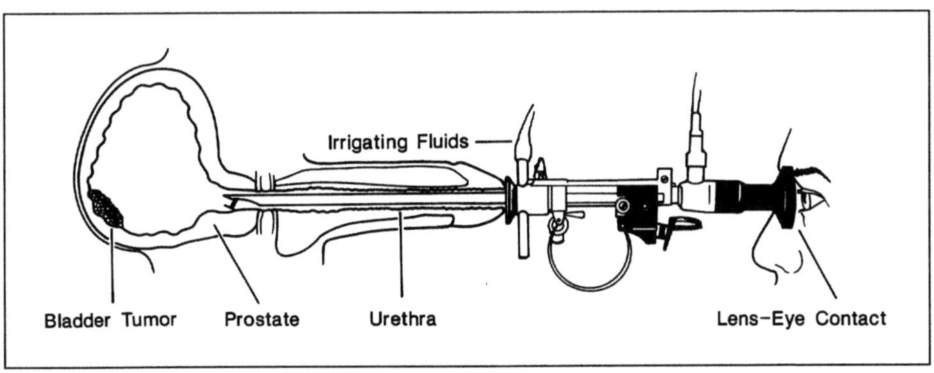

Fig. 6. Possible sources of infection during transurethral resection of the prostate.

With the implementation of video cameras and television screens to perform TURP, lens-eye contact is no longer necessary and may result in reduced infection rates. There must be a clear differentiation between patients with preoperatively infected urine and those with sterile urine. Bacteremia following TURP is a common finding, occurring in 11 % of patients with sterile urine (Biorn et al., 1950; Creevy and Feeny, 1954). However, if the urine is infected, positive blood cultures are found in 50 % (Sullivan et al., 1973). Preoperative bacteriuria is clearly a risk factor for post-operative septicemia (Adolfsson et al., 1989; Cafferkey et al., 1987; Haverkorn, 1984). Because TURP requires postoperative urethral catheterization and a UTI does not usually clear unless antimicrobials are applied (Gordon et al., 1983), it is generally agreed to treat any UTI before TURP is performed (Kaiser, 1986).

The question as to whether antimicrobials should be administered to patients with sterile urine who undergo TURP is controversial. In a review article, Chodak and Plaut (1979) were unable to draw definite conclusions as to the benefit of antimicrobial prophylaxis in urologic surgery, mainly because of the poor design of the studies reviewed. They called for prospective, randomized, controlled trials. Since then, many such studies have been published, but have not ended the dispute. Although it appears certain that many antimicrobials will reduce the incidence of bacteriuria postoperatively, this bacteriuria is mostly asymptomatic and harmless. Therefore, it could be argued that it is better to treat bacteriuria when it occurs than to prophylactically lower the incidence. This question is still unanswered and will probably remain so.

Table 5 lists selected studies on this matter published within the last twelve years. Inconsistencies exist among these studies regarding the definition of significant bacteriuria, but all patients cited had preoperative sterile urine and were evaluated between the fifth and seventh post-operative day.

Five studies found no effect of prophylaxis on the infection rate (Ferrie and Scott, 1984; Qvist et al., 1984; Millar et al., 1987; Stricker and Grant, 1988; Houle et al., 1989). This may well be for statistical reasons. It has been calculated that the studies by Ferrie and Qvist had a statistical power of < 50 %, indicating a 50 % chance of overlooking a significant difference between treatment and placebo groups (Gasser et al., 1987). The study by Houle et al. (1989) found an unmatched low bacteriuria number, even in the control group, which is not explained. The study by Millar et al. (1987) was well-designed and found no significant difference between the two groups. There was a clear trend toward fewer infections in the prophylaxis group. Stricker and Grant (1988) found no significant difference between the two groups. They found that a break in the closed drainage system was far more important than use of antimicrobials. Forty percent of the patients who developed a UTI had a break in the closed drainage system; this break occurred in 10 % of patients without postoperative UTI.

All of the other studies demonstrated statistically significant reductions in infection rate from approximately 30 % to well below 10 %, among them the ones using quinolones as the active agent (Ueda et al., 1991; Abbou et al., 1989). Even with every reasonable effort to identify bacteriuric patients preoperatively, up to 19 % will unknowingly be infected during surgery (Shearman, 1987), particularly in the case of preoperative indwelling catheters (Hansen et al., 1987). In a study that included these unsuspected cases, the treated patients fared significantly better than the nontreated patients with respect to febrile episodes, complications, and length of hospital stay (Hargreave et al., 1982). In another study, up to 21 % undergoing TURP for obstruction had a prostatic infection, placing them at high post-operative risk. However, 82 % of these patients had a sterile urine culture preoperatively (Gorelick et al., 1988). There have been indications that

Table 5. Controlled studies of antimicrobial prophylaxis in patients undergoing transurethral resection of the prostate.

Year	Series	Level of significant Bacteriuria (CFU/ml)	Number of Patients	Prophylaxis	Rate of Infection (%) Treated Patients	Rate of Infection (%) Control Patients
1980	Williams et al.	$>10^5$	135	Cephradine[a]	12	43[d]
1981	Nielsen et al.	$>10^5$	99	Cefoxitin[a]	7	42[d]
1983	Childs et al.	$>10^5$	92	Ceftriaxone[a]	5	30[d]
1983b	Goldwasser et al.	$>10^5$	81	Co-trimoxazole[a]	4	32[d]
1983	Falkiner et al.	$>10^5$	60	Nitrofurantoin[a]	7	48[d]
1984	Dörflinger & Madsen	$>10^5$	68	Cefoperazone[a]	0	17[d]
1984	Grabe et al.	$>10^7$	82	Cefotaxime[a]	5	40[d]
1984	Ferrie & Scott	$>10^8$	58	Cefuroxime[a]	4	6[e]
1984	Qvist et al.	$>10^5$	88	Cefotaxime[b]	13	19[e]
1985	Allan & Kumar	N/A[c]	100	Mezlozillin[b]	20	64[d]
1986	Prokocimer et al.	$>10^5$	90	Cefotaxime[a]	4	30
1987	Millar et al.	$>10^5$	179	Aztreonam[b]	22	32[d]
1987	Desai et al.	$>10^5$	80	Enoxacin[a]	8	38[d]
1988	Stricker & Grant	$>10^5$	93	Ampicillin/ Gentamicine[b]	17	16[e]
1988	Taylor et al.	$>10^5$	235	Temocillin[a]	13	24[d]
1989	Houle et al.	$>10^5$	110	Cefoperazone[a]	0	2[e]
1989	Kjaergard et al.	$>10^8$	131	Clindamycin/ Gentamicine[b]	12	36[d]
1989	Abbou et al.	$>10^5$	80	Pefloxacin[a]	5	33[d]
1991	Ueda et al.	$>10^4$	58	Ofloxacin[a]	27	56[d]
1992	Slavis et. al	$>10^4$	107	Cefonicid[b]	12	37[d]

[a] Administered perioperatively (before, during, and after surgery). [b] Administered preoperatively. [c]N/A = Information not available. [d] Significant difference. [e] Nonsignificant difference.

urethral stricture formation was higher in patients who did not receive antimicrobials (Grabe and Hellsten, 1985).

No evidence exists that short-term administration of prophylactic antimicrobials results in the development of resistant strains (Bentsi et al., 1987). Therefore, antimicrobial prophylaxis is recommended for patients with sterile urine who undergo TURP.

In addition to systemic antimicrobials, application of local antiseptics has been investigated. Bladder irrigation with chlorhexidine following transurethral operations reduced the incidence of postoperative bacteriuria from 37 % in control patients to 13 % in treated patients (Ball et al., 1987). However, preexisting infections were not eliminated by this regimen. Conversely, application of antiseptic lubricating jelly into the urethra was not effective in reducing postoperative bacteriuria (Prescott et al., 1990).

5.2.4. Transurethral resection of bladder tumors (TURB)

The information presented for TURP basically holds true for transurethral resection of the bladder (TURB). One study has reported that the incidence of post-operative bacteriuria following TURB is higher than after TURP (Appell et al., 1980), but another report found a lower incidence (Goldwasser et al., 1983a). Occult bacterial colonization of bladder tumors was confirmed in both reports, and therefore may be an additional source of infection. Consequently, antimicrobial prophylaxis is also suggested for patients with sterile urine who undergo TURB.

5.2.5. Ureterorenoscopy (URS)

Prophylactic studies exclusively about ureterorenoscopy (URS) do not exist. One study on endoscopic extraction of upper urinary tract stones included URS and percutaneous surgery (Fourcade et al., 1990). This study found a significant reduction in post-operative bacteriuria from 25 % in the placebo group to 8.5 % in the cefotaxime-treated group. As in any transurethral surgery, the scope must be passed through the urethra and the bladder into the ureter. Therefore, the same sources of infection as in TURP must be considered. Moreover, up to 70 % of branched renal calculi are infected despite sterile urine; therefore, antimicrobial prophylaxis appears to be particularly worthwhile in this group of patients (Fowler, 1984). Considering the high percentage of urease positive bacteria, the agent of choice should have an antimicrobial spectrum that covers these troublesome microorganisms.

5.2.6. Percutaneous surgery

Percutaneous nephrolitholapaxy (PNL) is another endoscopic operation to treat kidney stones (Brannen et al., 1985). No controlled studies addressing the use of systemic antimicrobial prophylaxis in percutaneous surgery have been published. However, one study comparing PNL and open surgery found no infectious complications of PNL as compared to 4 % wound infections in open surgery (Brannen et al., 1985). Another study compared nephrolithotomy and PNL and found a 10 % wound infection rate in nephrolithotomy patients and a 37 % UTI rate in PNL patients (Assimos et al., 1991). Serious infectious complications such as pyelonephritis (15 %) and sepsis (4 %) occurred in the PNL group, but not in the nephrolithotomy group. A study of 126 patients found a 35 % postoperative bacteriuria rate in the face of preoperatively sterile urine (Charton et al., 1986). Conversely, preoperative bacteriuria and pyuria represented a risk factor for postoperative bacteremia and endotoxemia in a study of 117 patients who underwent endourological manipulation for stones in the upper urinary tract (Rao et al., 1991). In this study, the infection risk in PNL was higher than in URS and ESWL.

A double-blind, randomized, placebo-controlled study using noxythiolin (a topical bactericidal agent) irrigation of the upper urinary tract found this regimen to be a beneficial adjunct to reducing infectious risk in patients undergoing percutaneous surgery (Buck, 1988). As there is always the possibility of bacteria harbored within the stone, antimicrobials should be given during a PNL.

New percutaneous surgical techniques include laparoscopic ligation of spermatic veins (Matsuda et al., 1992) and pelvic lymphadenectomy (Schuessler et al., 1991). Studies of infectious complications are not yet available, but so far, no infectious complications have been reported. As the endoscopic picture is transferred to a TV screen, direct contact between the endoscope and the eye of the surgeon is no longer necessary. If safe antiseptic rules are applied, this surgical procedure can be considered clean, and antimicrobials are probably not necessary.

5.3. Open Surgery

5.3.1. Surgery of kidneys and external genitalia

Surgical procedures of the kidneys such as nephrectomy, partial nephrectomy, and pyeloplasty are considered clean operations (Childs, 1983). While most surgeons would agree on administration of antimicrobials to patients with drainage tubes and catheters in place for a lengthy period of time (as in pyeloplasty), this may not be the case for simple nephrectomy.

Operations on external genitalia also have a low risk of infection, and antimicrobials may not be necessary. However, a large, prospective, randomized, placebo-controlled, double-blind cefonicid study, including clean operations such as mastectomy and herniorrhaphy, found a significant reduction in infectious complications in the treatment group (Platt et al., 1990). The reduction in wound infections was from 12.2 % to 6.2 % and from 4.2 % to 2.3 % for mastectomy and herniorrhaphy, respectively. This indicates that antimicrobial prophylaxis may also be worthwhile for clean operations. This is particularly true when a prosthetic device such as a penile prosthesis is introduced (Chao et al., 1991).

General agreement exists to institute antimicrobial prophylaxis on patients undergoing open renal surgery of kidney stones, as there is always the possibility of releasing bacteria trapped in the stones (Lewi et al., 1983; Harrison et al., 1977). Various antimicrobial regimens are effective in reducing UTI and wound infections following open surgery.

5.3.2. Open prostatectomy

By perfecting the transurethral technique, fewer open prostatectomies are performed to relieve prostatic obstruction. The suprapubic approach is used to enucleate large adenoma or for radical prostatectomy in localized prostatic cancer. In addition to the infection risk after TURP, retropubic prostatectomy includes the risk of osteitis pubis and wound infection (Hock and Kurtz, 1951; Meares, 1975). There are few recent studies on prophylaxis in open prostatectomies, as these operations are usually included in studies of TURP. In a review of 761 retropubic prostatectomies, Marshall (1967) found an overall postoperative infection rate of 23 % in patients with preoperative sterile urine, vs. 44 % in patients with preoperative bacteriuria. In a placebo-controlled trimethoprim study by Haverkorn (1984), 24 % of patients in the placebo group had positive blood cultures vs. 9 % in the treatment group. Williams et al. (1980) investigated 57 patients undergoing retropubic prostatectomy. In patients with preoperatively sterile urine, the placebo group had an infection rate of 42 % compared to 33 % of the cephradine-treated group. Again, in preoperatively bacteriuric patients, the post-operative infection risk rose to 71 % and 67 % in placebo and treatment groups, respectively. A recent study of 150 consecutive patients undergoing open prostatectomy found a wound infection rate of 23 % and 9 % in patients with infected and sterile urine, respectively (Richter et al., 1991). Despite antibiotic prophylaxis, the authors recommended that prostatectomy be deferred until urine becomes sterile. As the infection rate after open prostatectomy is as high as that following TURP, antimicrobial prophylaxis is recommended, based on the same principles as for TURP.

5.3.3. Cystectomy with urinary diversion

Cystectomy for treatment of bladder cancer requires some kind of urinary diversion. The diversion may be an ileal loop or one of the various pouches recently described (Marshall, 1991). However, the common denominator of all these surgical procedures is use of the small or large bowel to create the reservoir or the conduit. No studies have been published specifically about prophylaxis in urinary diversion. These operations have to be considered contaminated at least (National Research Council, 1964). Therefore, an antimicrobial regimen should be administered (as in colonic surgery) and should significantly reduce the rate of wound infection (Kaiser, 1986). This regimen should cover the anaerobic bacteria. Therefore, quinolones alone are not sufficient to provide protection and should be combined with antimicrobials that are active against anaerobic bacteria.

5.3.4. Kidney transplantation

A detailed discussion of infections occurring in the kidney transplant patient is beyond the scope of this article and has been extensively reviewed elsewhere (Rubin and Young, 1988). However, as many urologists are involved in the care of such patients, a short overview of the infections in kidney transplantation seems warranted.

As many as 80 % of renal transplant patients suffer at least one infection during the first year after surgery. Infections remain the leading cause of death (Barnes et al., 1975). Many of the these infections are viral or fungal in origin, but bacterial infections also pose a threat to the patient in the early days after transplantation (Rubin et al., 1981). Indeed, during the first month after transplantation, the major causes of infection are the bacterial wound, pulmonary and urinary tract infections, and intravenous catheter related infections. Prevention of such infections includes eradication of a smoldering bacterial infection before transplantation, as this infection may flare up during immunosuppression despite impeccable surgical technique, and antimicrobial administration. The incidence of wound infections was reported as 41 % of patients, with Gram-negative bacteria being responsible in 73 % of these cases (Burgos-Calderon et al., 1971). With the advent of newer, less aggressive immunosuppressive regimens, the wound infection dropped to 1.7 % in uncomplicated wounds, and to 18.5 % in a transplant wound reopened for reasons other than infection (Schweizer et al., 1973).

Diabetes and retransplantation are associated with increased risk of 6.1 % in wound infections (Kyriakides et al., 1975). Bacteremia is a frequent complication of kidney transplantation. In the early postoperative course, 50 % to 75 % of the patients develop significant bacteremia (Bennett et al., 1970; Ramsey et al., 1979). One study reported 53 episodes in 140 patients, with the urinary tract being the primary focus in 60 % (Myerowitz et al., 1972). Elective appendectomy performed at the time of transplantation has been associated with a high incidence of Bacteroides fragilis bacteremia (Fisher et al., 1981). Therefore, any elective surgery should be avoided at the time of transplantation.

Septicemia may have particularly severe consequences for transplant patients. While Candida septicemia is associated with metastatic infections in < 5 % of normal individuals, more than 50 % of immunosuppressed patients will develop metastatic infection if untreated (Vincenti et al., 1982).

Undoubtedly, as in other patients, an indwelling catheter represents the major risk factor for the development of UTI. Culturing the tip of indwelling catheters has not been useful in the normal host. One study of 61 transplant patients reported that 16/24 patients with positive tip cultures subsequently developed UTI; in contrast, none of 15 with negative tip cultures developed UTI (Burleson et al., 1977). Not only is bacteriuria associated with the risk of bacteremia, with more severe consequences in transplant patients, but there is a suggested association between UTI and graft rejection (Byrd et al., 1978). Therefore, prevention of post-operative infection in transplant patients includes many measures. Careful surgical technique becomes even more important than in other surgical areas. Any existing infection should be eradicated before transplantation, and unnecessary surgery should be avoided. Wound irrigation with topical antimicrobial agents prevents infection (Belzer et al., 1973). Urinary and intravenous catheters should be removed at the earliest possible time. Prophylactic antimicrobials are recommended in kidney transplantation. One study attributed the reduced wound infection rate and improved survival rate of the patients with the use of broad spectrum antimicrobials (Tilney et al., 1978). Another study demonstrated a complete elimination of UTI in the first four months after transplantation using long term, low dose antimicrobials, compared to 23 % in the control group (Lemmers and Barry, 1991).

5.4. Various Urologic Procedures

5.4.1. Biopsy of the prostate

5.4.1.1. Transrectal biopsy

Transrectal biopsy of the prostate is performed to obtain tissue for cytological or histological examination. With the advent of transrectal ultrasound, the frequency of transrectal biopsy has increased, especially with the use of smaller needles. Reported infectious complications following transrectal biopsy include UTI, bacteremia, fever, prostatitis, epididymitis, pyelonephritis, local abscess, and even osteomyelitis (Larsen et al., 1986; Crawford et al., 1982). Bacteremia has been reported in up to 70 % of patients following transrectal biopsy (Ruebush et al., 1979), but usually approximate 40 % (Fong et al., 1991; Sharpe et al., 1982; Crawford et al., 1982). The bacteriuria rate ranges between 21 % and 36 % (Crawford et al., 1982; Ruebush et al., 1979). Trimethoprim sulfamethoxazole did not reduce the rate of bacteremia in two studies, but significantly reduced fever in one of the studies. However, the rate of UTI was dramatically reduced below 2 %. The reported result for trimethoprim sulfamethoxazole was better than for a combination of netilmycin and metronidazole, or carbenicillin (Fong et al., 1991; Crawford et al., 1982). This may be due to better penetration of trimethoprim into the prostate (IV). Another recent study demonstrated a bacteremia rate of 7 % for ciprofloxacin treated patients vs. 37 % for gentamycin treated patients, suggesting that quinolones are a good choice for prophylaxis (Roach et al., 1991). Cleansing enemas containing povidone-iodine did not reduce the incidence of infectious complications as compared to saline irrigation (Sharpe et al., 1982).

In view of the results of these studies, systemic antimicrobials are recommended for patients undergoing core biopsy of the prostate. However, this may not be necessary for transrectal needle aspiration of the prostate with a very thin instrument. No studies addressing this question are available at present.

5.4.1.2. Transperineal biopsy

With further development of transrectal prostatic ultrasound, transperineal biopsy will be used less frequently. Transient bacteremia occurs in less than 10 %. In contrast to transrectal biopsy, it is usually not caused by anaerobic bacteria (Hillyard, 1987). One study of 162 patients found no difference between placebo and trimethoprim or cephalosporin with respect to febrile episodes and UTI (Packer et al., 1984). Therefore, in cases of preoperative sterile urine and adequate skin preparation, transperineal biopsy can be considered clean, and antimicrobial prophylaxis is not necessary.

5.4.2. Extracorporeal shock wave lithotripsy (ESWL)

Extracorporeal shock wave lithotripsy (ESWL) has revolutionized the treatment of kidney and ureteral stones. However, literature regarding infectious complications of ESWL is sparse. As urinary calculi may harbor bacteria at the surface (Fowler, 1984) or within the stone (Nickel et al., 1986), these bacteria may be released during ESWL. This could result in bacteriuria and bacteremia. However, in a study of 23 patients we found that bacteremia occurred in less than 5 % (Gasser and Frei, 1992). Bacteriuria has been found in 5 % of patients with preoperative sterile urine who undergo ESWL. This low incidence per se does not justify routine antimicrobial prophylaxis for every patient. However, one should always consider the possibility of obstruction due to passing fragments with subsequent infection. This calls for careful evaluation and surveillance of patients at risk. In a recent study of patients undergoing ESWL, 14 % had bacteremia (Müller-Mattheis et al., 1991). Therefore, patients at risk for subacute bacterial endocarditis should receive perioperative antimicrobial prophylaxis according to guidelines for the prevention of subacute bacterial endocarditis (Malinverni et al., 1984; Simmons et al., 1982).

5.5. Various High-Risk Conditions

Many of the conditions which place patients at increased risk for infection have been discussed in previous sections. One must distinguish between situational and individual characteristics that place these patients at increased risk of infection (Tables 6 and 7).

5.5.1. Situations predisposing to infection

The most important factor for wound infection is the classification of the wound as designated by the National Research Council (Table 2). Not surprisingly, the wound infection rate is highest in dirty wounds and lowest in clean wounds. Other factors associated with a high risk of wound infection are abdominal operations and procedures over 2 hours long (Haley et al., 1985a). The length of the preoperative hospital stay is directly correlated

Table 6. Situations placing patients at risk for infection. (Modified from Larsen et al., 1986)

Indwelling catheters
Infected roommate
Prolonged preoperative hospitalization
Preoperative shaving
Wound classification
Surgery
Poor technique
Contaminated equipment
Extensive blood loss
Improper drainage
Excessive cauterization
Necrotic debris
Prolonged surgery
Abdominal surgery

Table 7. Individual patient characteristics that increase risk of infection

Recurrent urinary tract infection
Pregnancy
Female
Older
Serious underlying disease
Diabetes mellitus
Immunosuppression
Obesity
Malnutrition
Remote infection
Cancer
Defective or artificial heart valve
Alcoholism

with the incidence of wound infection. Studies by the National Research Council (1964) and Cruse and Foord (1980) have consistently found a clean wound infection rate of 1 % after one preoperative hospital day; when this time period increased to one week and 2 weeks, the rate increased to 2 % and 4 %, respectively. Preoperative shaving may predispose the patient to wound infection, particularly if performed the day before surgery. The wound infection rate was 6 % in patients shaved the day before surgery, as compared to 1.9 % in patients shaved the day of surgery (Olson et al., 1984).

Not surprisingly, indwelling catheters are the single most influential risk factor for UTI development (Stamm et al., 1977). Eighty percent of all nosocomial UTI are related to catheterization. Other "non-patient" factors which determine infection risk include the surgeon's skill, amount of blood loss, and surgical postponement for administrative reasons. Improper use of drains and inadequately sized urethral catheters can affect drainage of blood and other body fluids, promoting environments which foster bacterial growth. Overuse of electrical cauterization in open or transurethral procedures, or failure to remove all necrotic debris such as prostatic chips may also promote infection.

5.5.2. Patient characteristics predisposing to infection

In general, females, older individuals, and those with a medical history of recurrent UTI or prostatitis, and pregnancy are at higher risk for infection (Haley et al., 1981a). Poor general health, as indicated by three or more underlying diseases, also represents a high risk situation (Haley et al., 1985b). Cancer patients undergoing chemotherapy are also at risk (Gross et al., 1980). In the study by the National Research Council, the overall wound infection rate rose from 7.1 % to 10.4 % in diabetic patients, was 16% in patients undergoing preoperative steroid therapy, 18.1 % in obese patients, and 22.4 % in patients with severe malnutrition. Similar percentages have been reported in the Foothill hospital study (Cruse and Foord, 1980). Immunocompromized patients are at risk for bacterial infection, particularly if the granulocyte count is below $1500/mm^3$ (Rubin and Young, 1988). This is also true for patients with hematologic disorders or Acquired immunodeficiency syndrome (AIDS). Patients with a daily alcohol consumption level of $\geq$ 60 g are at increased risk of infections, i.e., cystitis, epididymitis, or septicemia, following TURP (Tönnesen et al., 1988).

Patients with a defective or artificial heart valve are at high risk for subacute bacterial endocarditis, which often originates in the urogenital tract (Svanbom and Strandell, 1978). These patients require antimicrobial prophylaxis according to guidelines for prevention of subacute bacterial endocarditis (Malinverni et al., 1984; Simmons et al., 1982).

VI. Literature

Abbou, C., Chopin, D., Nguyen, M., Theodon, P., Antiphon, P., Goulois, R., Bouleau, D.: Short-term pefloxacin prophylaxis in transurethral resection of the prostate. Rev. Inf. Dis. 11 (suppl 5): 1361, 1989.

Adolfsson, J., Köhler, C., Falck, L.: Norfloxacin versus trimethoprim-sulfamethoxazole. A study in patients with known bacteriuria undergoing transurethral resection of the prostate. Scand. J. Urol. Nephrol. 23: 255-259, 1989.

Allais, J. M., Preheim, L. C., Cuevas, T. A., Roccaforte, J. S., Mellencamp, M. A., Bittner, M. J.: Randomized, double-blind comparison of ciprofloxacin and trimethoprim-sulfamethoxazole for complicated urinary tract infections. Antimicrob. Agents Chemother. 32: 1327-1330, 1988.

Allan, W. R., Kumar, A.: Prophylactic mezlocillin for transurethral prostatectomy. Br. J. Urol. 57: 46-49, 1985.

Andriole, V. T.: Use of quinolones in treatment of prostatitis and lower urinary tract infections. In: Proceedings 3rd International Symposium on New Quinolones, Vancouver, Canada, July 12-14, 1990. Eur. J. Clin. Microbiol. Infect. Dis.(special issue): 122-130, 1991.

Appell, R. A., Flynn, J. T., Paris, A. M. I., Blandy, J. P.: Occult bacterial colonization of bladder tumors. J. Urol. 124: 345-346, 1980.

Assimos, D. G., Wrenn, J. J., Harrison, L. H., McCullough, D. L., Boyce, W. H., Taylor, C. L., Zagoria, R. J., Dyer, R. B.: A comparison of anatropic nephrolithotomy and percutaneous nephrolithotomy with and without extracorporeal shock wave lithotripsy for management of patients with staghorn calculi. J. Urol. 145: 710-714, 1991.

Bagley, D. H., Herlihy, E., McGuire, E. J.: Infections and antibiotic prophylaxis in the fulgurated rat bladder. Invest. Urol. 17: 277-283, 1980.

Ball, A. J., Carr, T. W., Gillespie, W. A., Kelly, M., Simpson, R. A., Smith, P. J. B.: Bladder irrigation with chlorhexidine for the prevention of urinary infection after transurethral operations: A prospective controlled Study. J. Urol. 138: 491-494, 1987.

Barbalias, G. A., Meares, E. M., Sant G. R.: Prostatodynia: Clinical and urodynamic characteristics. J. Urol. 130: 514-517, 1983

Barnes, B. A., Bergan, J. J., Braun, W. E., Fraumeni, J. F. Jr., Kountz, S. L., Mickey, M. R., Rubin, A. L., Simmons, R. L., Stevens, L. E., Wilson, R. E.: The 12th report of the human renal transplant registry. JAMA 233: 787-796, 1975.

Barrington, F. J. F., Wright, H. D.: Bacteriaemia following operations on the urethra. J. Pathol. Bacteriol. 33: 871-888, 1930.

Belzer, F. O., Salvatierra, O., Schweizer, R. T., Kountz, S. L.: Prevention of wound infections by topical antibiotics in high risk patients. Am. J. Surg. 126: 180-185, 1973.

Bennett, W. M., Beck, C. H. Jr., Young, H. H., Russell, P. S.: Bacteriuria in the first month following renal transplantation. Arch. Surg. 101: 453-456, 1970.

Bentsi, I. K., Elton, R. A., Ritchie, A. W. S., Smith, G., Gould, J. C., Chisholm, G. D., Hargreave, T. B.: Antibiotic prophylaxis for prostatic surgery. Single-dose cephradine compared with single-dose cefotaxime. Br. J. Urol. 59: 314-318, 1987.

Berger, R. E., Krieger, J. N., Kessler, D., Ireton, R. C., Close, C., Holmes, K. K., Roberts, P. L.: Case-control study of men with suspected chronic idiopathic prostatitis. J. Urol. 141: 328-331, 1989.

Biorn, C. L., Browning, W. H., Thompson, L.: Transient bacteremia immediately following transurethral prostatic resection. J. Urol. 63: 155-161, 1950.

Boerema, J. B. J., Dalhoff, A., Debruyne, F. M. Y.: Ciprofloxacin distribution in prostatic tissue and fluid following oral administration. Chemotherapy 31: 13-18, 1985.

Brannen, G. E., Bush, W. H., Correa, R. J., Gibbons, R. P., Elder, J. S.: Kidney stone removal: Percutaneous versus surgical lithotomy. J. Urol. 133: 6-12, 1985.
Brehmer, B., Madsen, P. O.: Route and prophylaxis of ascending bladder infection in male patients with indwelling catheters. J. Urol. 108: 719-721, 1972.
Brumfitt, W., Smith, G., Hamilton-Miller, J. M. T.: Norfloxacin vs. macrodantin for the prophylaxis of recurrent urinary tract infection in women. Rev. Infect. Dis. 11 (suppl 5): 1338, 1989.
Bryan, C. S., Reynolds, K. L.: Hospital-acquired bacteremic urinary tract infection: Epidemiology and outcome. J. Urol. 132: 494-498, 1984.
Buck, A. C.: The use of noxythiolin (noxyflex 'S') as an antiseptic irrigant in upper urinary tract drainage following percutaneous nephrolithotomy. Br. J. Urol. 62: 306-310, 1988.
Burgos-Calderon, R., Pankey, G. A., Figueroa, J. E.: Infection in kidney transplatation. Surgery 70: 334-340, 1971.
Burke, J. F.: The effective period of preventive antibiotic action in experimental incisions and dermal lesions. Surgery 50: 161-168, 1961.
Burke, J. P., Garibaldi, R. A., Britt, M. R., Jacobson, J. A., Conti, M., Alling, D. W.: Prevention of catheter-associated urinary tract infections. Am. J. Med. 70: 655-658, 1981.
Burleson, R. L., Brennan, A. M., Scruggs, B. F.: Foley catheter tip cultures. A valuable diagnostic aid in the immunosuppressed patient. Am. J. Surg. 133: 723-725, 1977.
Byrd, L. H., Tapia, L., Cheigh, J. S., Aronian, J., Stenzel, K. H., Rubin, A. I.: Association between streptococcus faecalis urinary infections and graft rejection in kidney transplantation. Lancet ii: 1167-1169, 1978.
Cafferkey, M. T., Falkiner, F. R., Gillespie, W. A., Murphy, D. M.: Antibiotics for the prevention of septicaemia in urology. J. Antimicrob. Chemother. 9: 471-477, 1982.
Chao, R., Bejany, D. E., Politano, V. A., Rhamy, R. K., Aviles, A.: Oral ciprofloxacin prophylaxis in the insertion of penile prosthesis. J. Urol. 145 (suppl): 238A, 1991.
Charton, M., Vallancien, G., Veillon, B., Brisset, J. M.: Urinary tract infection in percutaneous surgery for renal calculi. J. Urol. 135: 15-17, 1986.
Childs, S. J.: Genitourinary surgical prophylaxis. Infect. Surg. 2: 701-710, 1983.
Childs, S. J., Wells, W. G., Mirelman, S.: Antibiotic prophylaxis for genitourinary surgery in community hospitals. J. Urol. 130: 305-308, 1983.
Chodak, G. W., Plaut, M. E.: Systemic antibiotics for prophylaxis in urologic surgery: A critical review. J. Urol. 121: 695-699, 1979.
Classen, D. C., Evans, R. S., Pestotnik, S. L., Horn, S. D., Menlove, R. L., Burke, J. P.: The timing of prophylactic administration of antibiotics and the risk of surgical-wound infection. N. Engl. J. Med. 326: 281-286, 1992.
Classen, D. C., Larsen, R. A., Burke, J. P., Alling, D. W., Stevens, L. E.: Daily meatal care for prevention of catheter-associated bacteriuria: Results using frequent applications of polyantibiotic cream. Infect. Control Hosp. Epidemiol. 12: 157-162, 1991.
Cohen, A.: A microbiological comparison of povidone-iodine lubricating gel and a control as catheter lubricants. J. Hosp. Infect. 6 (suppl): 155-161, 1985.
Cox, C. E.: Ofloxacin in the management of complicated urinary tract infections, including prostatitis. Am. J. Med. 87 (suppl 6C): 61-68, 1989.
Crawford, E. D., Haynes, A. L., Story, M. W., Borden, T. A.: Prevention of urinary tract infection and sepsis following transrectal prostatic biopsy. J. Urol. 127: 449-451, 1982.
Creevy, C. D., Feeny, M. J.: Routine use of antibiotics in transurethral prostatic resection: A clinical investigation. J. Urol 71: 615-623, 1954.
Cruse, P. J. E., Foord, R.: The epidemiology of wound infection. A 10-year prospective study of 62,939 wounds. Surg. Clin. N. Am. 60: 27-40, 1980.
Desai, K. M., Abrams, P. H., White, L. O.: A double-blind comparative trial of short-term orally administered enoxacin in the prevention of urinary infection after elective transurethral prostatectomy: A clinical and pharmacokinetic study. J. Urol. 139: 1232-1235, 1988.
Doble, A., Thomas, B. J., Walker, M. M., Harris, J. R. W., Witherow, R. O'N., Taylor-Robinson, D.: The role of chlamydia trachomatis in chronic abacterial prostatitis: A study using ultrasound guided biopsy. J. Urol. 141: 332-333, 1989.
Dörflinger, T., Madsen, P. O.: Antibiotic prophylaxis in transurethral surgery. Urology 24: 643-648, 1984.

Drach, T. U., Meares, E. M. Jr., Fair, W. R., Stamey, T. A.: Classification of benign diseases associated with prostatic pain: Prostatitis and prostatodynia. J. Urol. 120: 266, 1978.
Edwards, L. D.: The epidemiology of 2056 remote site infections and 1966 surgical wound infections occurring in 1865 Patients: A four year study of 40,923 operations at Rush-Presbyterian-St. Luke's Hospital, Chicago. Ann. Surg. 184: 758-767, 1976.
Ellner, P. D., Neu, H. C.: The inhibitory quotient. A method for interpreting minimum inhibitory concentration data. JAMA 246: 1575-1578, 1981.
Falkiner, F. R., Ma, P. T. S., Murphy, D. M., Cafferkey, M. T, Gillespie, W. A.: Antimicrobial agents for the prevention of urinary tract infection in transurethral surgery. J. Urol. 129: 766-768, 1983.
Fang, L. S. T, Tolkoff-Rubin, N. E., Rubin, R. H.: Efficacy of single-dose and conventional amoxicillin therapy in urinary tract infection localized by the antibody-coated bacteria technic. N. Engl. J. Med. 298: 413-416, 1978.
Ferrie, B. G., Scott, R.: Prophylactic cefuroxime in transurethral resection. Urol. Res. 12: 279-281, 1984.
Fisher, M. C., Baluarte, H. J., Long, S. S.: Bacteremia due to bacteroides fragilis after elective appendectomy in renal transplant recipients. J. Infect. Dis. 143: 635-638, 1981.
Fong, I. W., Struthers, N., Honey, R. J., Simbul, M., Boisseau, D. A.: A randomized comparative study of the prophylactic use of trimethoprim-sulfamethoxazole versus netilmycin-metronidazole in transrectal prostatic biopsy. J. Urol. 146: 794-797, 1991.
Fourcade, R. O. and the Cefotaxime Cooperative Group: Antibiotic prophylaxis with cefotaxime in endoscopic extraction of upper urinary tract stones: A randomized study. J. Antimicrob. Chemother. 26 (suppl A): 77-83, 1990.
Fowler, J. E.: Nosocomial catheter-associated urinary tract infection. Infect. Surg. 2: 43-53, 1983.
Fowler, J. E.: Bacteriology of branched renal calculi and accompanying urinary tract infection. J. Urol. 131: 213-215, 1984.
Garibaldi, R. A, Burke, J. P., Dickman, M. L., Smith, C. B.: Factors predisposing to bacteriuria during indwelling urethral catheterization. N. Engl. J. Med. 291: 215-219, 1974.
Garibaldi, R. A., Burke, J. P., Britt, M. R., Miller, W. A., Smith, C. B.: Meatal colonization and catheter-associated bacteriuria. N. Engl. J. Med. 303: 316-318, 1980.
Gasser, T. C., Graversen, P. H., Madsen, P. O.: Antimicrobial prophylaxis in surgery. N. Engl. J. Med. 316: 1089, 1987.
Gasser, T. C., Frei R.: Low bacteremia risk during extracorporeal shock wave lithotripsy. Br. J. Urol. (in press)
Gasser, T. C., Madsen, P. O.: Influence of urological irrigation fluids on urothelial bacterial adherence. (submitted for publication).
Gerding, D. N., Hitt, J. A.: Tissue penetration of the new quinolones in humans. Rev. Inf. Dis. 11 (suppl 5): S1046-S1057, 1989.
Goldwasser, B., Bogokowsky, B., Nativ, O., Sidi, A. A., Jonas, P., Many, M.: Urinary infections following transurethral resection of bladder tumors - rate and source. J. Urol. 129: 1123-1124, 1983a.
Goldwasser, B., Sidi, A. A., Bogokowsky, B., Jonas, P., Nativ, O., Many, M.: Prophylactic antimicrobial treatment in transurethral prostatectomy. How long should it be instituted? Urology 22: 136-138, 1983b.
Gordon, D. L., McDonald, P. J., Bune, A., Marshall, V. R., Grime, B., Marsh, J., Sinclair, G.: Diagnostic criteria and natural history of catheter-associated urinary tract infections after prostatectomy. Lancet ii: 1269-1271, 1983.
Gorelick, J. I., Senterfit, L. B., Vaughan, E. D. Jr.: Quantitative bacterial tissue cultures from 209 prostatectomy specimens: Findings and implications. J. Urol. 139: 57-60, 1988.
Grabe, M.: Antimicrobial agents in transurethral prostatic resection. J. Urol. 138: 245-252, 1987.
Grabe, M., Forsgren, A., Hellsten, S.: The effect of a short antibiotic course in transurethral prostatic resection. Scand. J. Urol. Nephrol. 18: 37-42, 1984.
Grabe, M., Hellsten, S.: Long-term follow-up after transurethral prostatic resection with or without a short peri-operative antibiotic course. Br. J. Urol. 57: 444-449, 1985.
Gross, P. A., Neu, H. C., Aswapokee, P., Van Antwerpen, C., Aswapokee, N.: Deaths from nosocomial infections: Experience in a university hospital and a community hospital. Am. J. Med. 68: 219-223, 1980.
Guglielmo, K. J., Hohn, D. C., Koo, P. J., Hunt, T. K., Sweet, R. L., Conte, J. E. Jr.: Antibiotic prophylaxis in surgical procedures. Arch. Surg. 118: 943-955, 1983.

Haase, D. A., Harding, G. K. M., Thomson, M. J., Kennedy, J. K., Urias, B. A., Ronald, A. R.: Comparative trial of norfloxacin and trimethoprim-sulfamethoxazole in the treatment of women with localized, acute, symptomatic urinary tract infections and antimicrobial effect on periurethral and fecal microflora. Antimicrob. Agents Chemother. 26: 481-484, 1984.

Haley, R. W., Culver, D. H., Morgan, W. M., White, J. W., Emori, T. G., Hooton, T. M.: Identifying patients at high risk of surgical wound infection. A Simple multivariate index of patient susceptibility and wound contamination. Am. J. Epidemiol. 121: 206-215, 1985a.

Haley, R. W., Culver, D. H., White, J. W., Morgan, W. M., Emori, T. G.: The nationwide nosocomial infection rate. A new need for vital statistics. Am. J. Epidemiol. 121: 159-167, 1985b.

Haley, R. W., Hooton, T. M., Culver, D. H., Stanley, R. C., Emori, T. G., Hardison, C. D., Quade, D., Shachtman, R. H., Schaberg, D. R., Shah, B. V., Schatz, G. D.: Nosocomial infections in U.S. hospitals, 1975-1976. Estimated frequency by selected characteristics of patients. Am. J. Med. 70: 947-959, 1981a.

Haley, R. W., Schaberg, D. R., Crossley, K. B., von Allmen, S. D., McGowan, J. E.: Extra charges and prolongation of stay attributable to nosocomial infections: A prospective interhospital comparison. Am. J. Med. 70: 51-58, 1981b.

Hansen, M., Genster, H. G., Thordsen, C.: Urinary tract infections in connection with transurethral resection of the prostate. Scand. J. Urol. Nephrol. 104: 65-68, 1987.

Hargreave, T. B., Hindmarsh, J. R., Elton, R., Chisholm, G. D., Gould, J. C.: Short-term prophylaxis with cefotaxime for prostatic surgery. Br. Med. J. 284: 1008-1010, 1982.

Harrison, L. H., Whitehurst, A. W., Boyce, W. H.: Adjuvant antimicrobial therapy with renal calculus surgery. J. Urol. 118: 233-236, 1977.

Hart, A. J. L., Miles, R. S., Varnam, D. J., Edmond, P.: Assessment of the morbidity and value of prophylactic cephazolin sodium in urinary tract instrumentation in out-patients. Curr. Med. Res. Opin. 6: 658-662, 1980.

Haverkorn, M. J.: Prophylactic trimethoprim for prostatectomy. Urology 24: 414-418, 1984.

Hillyard, J. W.: Bacteraemia following perineal prostatic biopsy. Br. J. Urol. 60: 252-254, 1987.

Hock, E. F., Kurtz, K. A.: Osteitis pubis. J. Urol. 65: 419-426, 1951.

Höffken, G., Lode, H., Prinzing, C., Borner, K., Koeppe, P.: Pharmacokinetics of ciprofloxacin after oral and parenteral administration. Antimicrob. Agents Chemother. 27: 375-379, 1985.

Holliman, R., Seal, D. V., Archer, H., Doman, S.: Controlled trial of chemical disinfection of urinary drainage bags. Reduction in hospital-acquired catheter-associated infection. Br. J. Urol. 60: 419-422, 1987.

Hooper, D. C., Wolfson, J. S.: Fluoroquinolone antimicrobial agents. N. Engl. J. Med. 324: 384-394, 1991.

Houle, A. M., Mokhless, I., Sarto, N., Elhilali, M. M.: Perioperative antibiotic prophylaxis for transurethral resection of the prostate: Is it justifiable? J. Urol. 142: 317-319, 1989.

Iversen, P., Madsen, P. O.: Bacterial adherence to urothelium following bladder irrigation in the rat. Infection 10: 116-119, 1982.

Kaiser, A. B.: Antimicrobial prophylaxis in surgery. N. Engl. J. Med. 315: 1129-1138, 1986.

Kass, E. H., Schneiderman, L. J.: Entry of bacteria into the urinary tracts of patients with inlying catheters. N. Engl. J. Med. 256: 556-557, 1957.

Kass, E. H.: The Role of asymptomatic bacteriuria in the pathogenesis of pyleonephritis. In: Quinn, E. L. and Kass, E. H.: Biology of pyleonephritis, Little Brown and Co., Boston, 1960.

Kjaergaard, B., Petersen, E., Lauridsen, K. G., Petersen, A. S.: Prophylactic one-dose treatment with clindamycin and gentamicin in transurethral prostatic resection. A double-blind placebo controlled study. Scand. J. Urol. Nephrol. 23: 109-113, 1989.

Korbel, E. I., Maher, P. O.: Use of prophylactic antibiotics in urethral instrumentation. J. Urol. 116: 744-746, 1976.

Kresken, M., Wiedemann, B.: Development of resistance to naldixic acid and the fluoroquinolones after the introduction of norfloxacin and ofloxacin. Antimicrob. Agents Chemother. 32: 1285-1288, 1988.

Krieger, J. N., Kaiser, D. L., Wenzel, R. P.: Nosocomial urinary tract infections: Secular trends, treatment and economics in a university hospital. J. Urol. 130: 102-106, 1983.

Kunin, C. M., Johansen, K. S., Worning, A. M., Daschner, F. D.: Report of a symposium on use and abuse of antibiotics worldwide. Rev. Inf. Dis. 12: 12-19, 1990.

Kunin, C. M., McCormack, R. C.: Prevention of catheter-induced urinary-tract infections by sterile closed drainage. N. Engl. J. Med. 274: 1155-1161, 1966.

Kyriakides, G. K., Simmons, R. L., Najarian, J. S.: Wound infections in renal transplant wounds: Pathogenetic and prognostic factors. Ann. Surg. 182: 770-775, 1975.

Lapides, J., Diokno, A. C., Lowe, B. S., Kalish, M. D.: Followup on unsterile intermittent self-catheterization. J. Urol. 111: 184-187, 1974.

Larsen, E. H., Gasser, T. C., Madsen, P. O.: Antimicrobial prophylaxis in urologic surgery. Urol. Clin. N. Am. 13: 591-604, 1986.

Ledergerber, B., Bettex, J.-D., Joos, B., Flepp, M., Lüthy, R.: Effect of standard breakfast on drug absorption and multiple-dose pharmacokinetics of ciprofloxacin. Antimicrob. Agents Chemother. 27: 350-352, 1985.

Lemmers, M. J., Barry, J. M.: Prophylaxis against urinary tract infections after renal transplantation: A randomized, prospective study. J. Urol. 145 (suppl 4): 346A, 1991.

Leport, C., Rousseau, F., Perronne, C., Salmon, D., Joerg, A., Vilde, J. L.: Bacterial prostatitis in patients infected with the human immunodeficiency virus. J. Urol. 141: 334-336, 1989.

Lewi, H. J. E., Hales, D. S. M., Ferguson, M., Wright, P. A., Scott, R.: Short course netilmicin prophylaxis in renal stone surgery. Urol. Res. 11: 207-210, 1983.

Maizels, M., Schaeffer, A. J.: Decreased incidence of bacteriuria associated with periodic instillations of hydrogen peroxide into the urethral catheter drainage bag. J. Urol. 123: 841-845, 1980.

McEniry, D. W., Gorbach, S. L.: Cephalosporins in surgery. Prophylaxis and therapy. Drugs 34 (suppl 2): 216-239, 1987.

McKittrick, L. S., Wheelock, F. C. Jr.: The routine use of antibiotics in elective abdominal surgery. Surg. Gynecol. Obstet. 99: 376-377, 1954.

Madsen, P. O., Dörflinger, T., Larsen, E. H., Gasser, T. C.: Pharmacokinetics of antibacterial agents used for the treatment of bacterial prostatitis. In: Weidner, W., et al. (ed.): Therapy of prostatitis. Experimental and clinical data. Zuckschwerdt, München: 17-20, 1986.

Malinverni, R., Francioli, P., Gerber, A., Glauser, M. P., Hirschel, B., Lüthy, R., Mombelli, G., Regamey, C., Schaad, U. B., Schädelin, J., Stalder, H., Zimmerli, W.: Prophylaxe der bakteriellen Endokarditis. Empfehlungen der Schweizerischen Arbeitsgruppe für Endokarditisprophylaxe. Schweiz. med. Wschr. 114: 1246-1252, 1984.

Manson, A. L.: Is antibiotic administration indicated after outpatient cystoscopy. J. Urol. 140: 316-317, 1988.

Marshall, A.: Retropubic prostatectomy: A review with special reference to urinary infection. Br. J. Urol. 39: 307-327, 1967.

Marshall, F. F. (Ed): Partial and total bladder reconstruction. Urol. Clin. N. Am. 18 (4), 1991.

Matsuda, T., Horii, Y., Higashi, S., Oishi, K., Takeuchi, H., Yoshida, O.: Laparoscopic varicocelectomy: A simple technique for clip ligation of the spermatic vessels. J. Urol. 147: 636-638, 1992.

Meares, E. M.: Factors that influence surgical wound infections. Role of prophylactic antibiotic therapy. Urology 6: 535-546, 1975.

Meares, E. M.: Prostatitis syndromes: New perspectives about old woes. J. Urol. 123: 141-147, 1980.

Meares, E. M., Stamey, T. A.: Bacteriological localization patterns in bacterial prostatitis and urethritis. Invest. Urol. 5: 492-518, 1968.

Michelson, J. D., Lotke, P. A., Steinberg, M. E.: Urinary-bladder management after total joint-replacement surgery. N. Engl. J. Med. 319: 321-326, 1988.

Millar, M. R., Inglis, T., Ewing, R., Clark, P., Williams, R. E., Lacey, R. W.: Double-blind study comparing aztreonam with placebo for prophylaxis of infection following prostatic surgery. Br. J. Urol. 60: 345-348, 1987.

Morris, M. J., Golovsky, D., Guinness, M. D. G., Maher, P. O.: The value of prophylactic antibiotics in transurethral prostatic resection: A controlled trial, with observations on the origin of postoperative infection. Br. J. Urol. 48: 479-484, 1976.

Mountokalakis, T., Skounakis, M., Tselentis, J.: Short-term versus prolonged systemic antibiotic prophylaxis in patients treated with indwelling catheters. J. Urol. 134: 506-508, 1985.

Müller-Mattheis, V. G. O., Schmale, D., Seewald, M., Rosin, H., Ackermann, R.: Bacteremia during extracorporeal shock wave lithotripsy of renal calculi. J. Urol. 146: 733-736, 1991.

Murdoch, D. A., Badenoch, D. F.: Oral ciprofloxacin as prophylaxis for optical urethrotomy. Br. J. Urol. 60: 352-354, 1987.

Myerowitz, R. L., Medeiros, A. A., O'Brian, T. F.: Bacterial infection in renal homotransplant recipients. A study of fifty-three bacteremic episodes. Am. J. Med. 53: 308-314, 1972.

Naber, K. G.: Use of quinolones in urinary tract infections and prostatitis. Rev. Inf. Dis. 11 (suppl 5): 1321-1337, 1989.

National Research Council: Postoperative wound infections. The influence of ultraviolet irradiation of the operating room and of various other factors. Ann. Surg. 160 (suppl 1): 1-192, 1964.

Nickel, J. C., Downey, J., Costerton, J. W.: Movement of pseudomonas aeruginosa along catheter surfaces. Urology 34: 93-98, 1992.

Nickel, J. C., Reid, G., Bruce, A. W., Costerton, J. W.: Ultrastructural microbiology of infected urinary stone. Urology 28: 512-515, 1986.

Nielsen, K. T., Madsen, P. O.: Quinolones in urology. Urol. Res. 17: 117-124, 1989.

Nielsen, O. S., Maigaard, S., Frimodt-Möller, N., Madsen, P. O.: Prophylactic antibiotics in transurethral prostatectomy. J. Urol. 126: 60-62, 1981.

Nielsen, O. S., Madsen, P. O.: Importance and timing of prophylactic antibiotics in urology with a special reference to growth and kill rates of E. coli in genitourinary organs. J. Urol. 128: 608-614, 1982.

Olson, M., O'Connor, M., Schwartz, M. L.: Surgical wound infections. A 5-Year prospective study of 20,193 wounds at the Minneapolis VA Medical Center. Ann. Surg. 199: 253-259, 1984.

Packer, M. G., Russo, P., Fair, W. R.: Prophylactic antibiotics and Foley catheter use in transperineal needle biopsy of the prostate. J. Urol. 131: 687-689, 1984.

Paquin, J. M., Perreault, J. P., Faucher, R., Mauffette, F., Valiquette, L., Lapointe, S.: Complications immédiates de la résection transurétrale de la prostate: Étude de 1000 cas consécutifs. Can. J. Surg. 31: 438-440, 1988.

Platt, R., Polk, B. F., Murdock, B., Rosner, B.: Mortality associated with nosocomial urinary-tract infection. N. Engl. J. Med. 307: 637-642, 1982.

Platt, R., Zaleznik, D. F., Hopkins, C. C., Dellinger, E. P., Karchmer, A. W., Bryan, C. S., Burke, J. F., Wikler, M. A., Marino, S. K., Holbrook, K. F., Tosteson, T. D., Segal, M. R.: Perioperative antibiotic prophylaxis for herniorrhaphy and breast surgery. N. Engl. J. Med. 322: 153-160, 1990.

Preheim, L. C., Cuevas, T. A., Roccaforte, J. S., Mellencamp, M. A., Bittner, M. J.: Ciprofloxacin and antacids. Lancet ii, 48, 1986.

Prescott, S., Hadi, M. A., Elton, R. A., Ritchie, A. W. S., Foubister, G. C., Gould, J. C., Hargreave, T. B.: Antibiotic compared with antiseptic prophylaxis for prostatic surgery. Br. J. Urol. 66: 509-514, 1990.

Prokocimer, P., Quazza, M., Gibert, C., Lemoine, J. E., Joly, M. L., Dureuil, B., Moulonguet, A., Manuel, C., Desmonts, J. M.: Short-term prophylactic antibiotics in patients undergoing prostatectomy: Report of a double-blind randomized trial with 2 intravenous doses of cefotaxime. J. Urol. 135: 60-64, 1986.

Qvist, N., Christiansen, H. M., Ehlers, D.: Prophylactic antibiotics in transurethral surgery. Urol. Res. 12: 275-277, 1984.

Ramsey, D. E., Finch, W. T., Birtch, A. G.: Urinary tract infections in kidney transplant recipients. Arch. Surg. 114: 1022-1025, 1979.

Rao, P. N., Dube, D. A., Weightman, N. C., Oppenheim, B. A., Morris, J.: Prediction of septicemia following endourological manipulation for stones in the upper urinary tract. J. Urol. 146: 955-960, 1991.

Reilly, C. S., Hart, A. J. L., McAllister, T. A.: Comparison of cephazolin and gentamicin in the prophylactic treatment of infection in out-patient urinary tract endoscopy. Br. J. Urol. 53: 138-140, 1981.

Richter, S., Lang, R., Zur, F., Nissenkorn, I.: Infected urine as a risk factor for postprostatectomy wound infection. Infect. Control. Hosp. Epidemiol. 12: 147-149, 1991.

Roach, M. B., George, W. J., Figueroa, T. E., Neal, D. E., McBride, D.: Ciprofloxacin versus gentamicin in prophylaxis against bacteremia in transrectal prostate needle biopsy. Urology 38: 84-87, 1991.

Rubin, R. H., Wolfson, J. S., Cosimi, A. B., Tolkoff-Rubin, N. E.: Infection in the renal transplant recipient. Am. J. Med. 70: 405-411, 1981.

Rubin, R. H., Young, L. S. (Eds.): Clinical approach to infection in the compromised host. Second Edition, Plenum Medical Book Co. New York, London, 1988.

Ruebush, T. K., McConville, J. H., Calia, F. M.: A double-blind study of trimethoprim-sulfamethoxazole prophylaxis in patients having transrectal needle biopsy of the prostate. J. Urol. 122: 492-494, 1979.

Rutledge, K. A., McDonald, H. P. Jr.: Costs of treating simple nosocomial urinary tract infection. Urology 26 (suppl): 24-26, 1985.

Rutkow, I. M.: Rates of surgery in the United States. Surg. Clin. N. Am. 62: 559-578, 1982.

Rutkow, I. M.: Urological operations in the United States: 1979 to 1984. J. Urol. 135: 1206-1208, 1986.

Sanchez-Ubeda, R., Fernand, E., Rousselot, L.M.: Complication rate in general surgical cases. N. Engl. J. Med. 259: 1045-1050, 1958.

Schaeffer, A. J., Sisney, G. A.: Efficacy of norfloxacin in urinary tract infections: Biological effects on vaginal and fecal flora. J. Urol. 133: 628-630, 1985.

Scheckler, W. E., Bennett, J. V.: Antibiotic usage in seven community hospitals. JAMA 213: 264-267, 1970.

Schuessler, W. W., Vancaillie, T. G., Reich, H., Griffith, D. P.: Transperitoneal endosurgical lymphadenectomy in patients with localized prostatic cancer. J. Urol. 145: 988-991, 1991.

Schweizer, R. T., Kountz, S. L., Belzer, F. O.: Wound complications in recipients of renal transplants. Ann. Surg. 177: 58-62, 1973.

Shapiro, J., Hoffmann, J., Jersky, J.: A comparison of suprapubic and transurethral drainage for postoperative urinary retention in general surgical patients. Acta. Chir. Scand. 148: 323-327, 1982.

Sharpe, J. R., Sadlowski, R. W., Finney, R. P., Branch, W. T., Hanna, J. E.: Urinary tract infection after transrectal needle biopsy of the prostate. J. Urol. 127: 255-256, 1982.

Shearman, C. P.: Antibiotic prophylaxis in transurethral prostatectomy. Br. J. Surg. 74: 653, 1987.

Simmons, N. A., Cawson, R. A., Clarke, C., Eykyn, S. J., McGowan, D. A., Oakley, C. M., Shanson, D. C.: The antibiotic prophylaxis of infective endocarditis. Report of a working party of the British society for antimicrobial chemotherapy. Lancet ii: 1323-1326, 1982.

Slavis, A. S., Miller, J. B., Golji, H., Dunshee, C. J.: Comparison of single-dose antibiotic prophylaxis in uncomplicated transurethral resection of the prostate. J. Urol. 147: 1303-1306, 1992

Stamey, T. A., Meares, E. M., Winningham, D. G.: Chronic bacterial prostatitis and the diffusion of drugs into prostatic fluid. J. Urol. 103: 187-194, 1970.

Stamm, W. E., Martin, S. M., Bennett, J. V.: Epidemiology of nosocomial infections due to gram-negative bacilli: Aspects revelant to development and use of vaccines. J. Infect. Dis. 136 (suppl): S151-S160, 1977.

Stark, R. P., Maki, D. G.: Bacteriuria in the catheterized patient. What quantitative level is significant? N. Engl. J. Med. 311: 560-564, 1984.

Stein, G. E., Mummaw, N., Goldstein, E. J. C., Boyko, E. J., Reller, L. B., Kurtz, T. O., Miller, K., Cox, C. E.: A multicenter comparative trial of three-day norfloxacin vs ten-day sulfamethoxazole and trimethoprim for the treatment of uncomplicated urinary tract infections. Arch. Intern. Med. 147: 1760-1762, 1987.

Stricker, P. D., Grant, A. B. F.: Relative value of antibiotics and catheter care in the prevention of urinary tract infection after transurethral prostatic resection. Br. J. Urol. 61: 494-497, 1988.

Sullivan, N. M, Sutter, V. L., Mims, M. M., Marsh, V. H., Finegold, S. M.: Clinical aspects of bacteremia after manipulation of the genitourinary tract. J. Infect. Dis. 127: 49-55, 1973.

Svanbom, M., Strandell, T.: Bacterial endocarditis. A prospective study of etiology, underlying factors and foci of infection. Scand. J. Infect. Dis. 10: 193-202, 1978.

Svanborg Edén, C., Hanson, L. A., Jodal, U., Lindeberg, U., Sohl Akerlund, A.: Variable adherence to normal human urinary-tract epithelial cells of Escherichia coli strains associated with various forms of urinary-tract infection. Lancet ii: 490-492, 1976.

Tartaglione, T. A., Raffalovich, A. C., Poynor, W. J., Espinel-Ingroff, A., Kerkering, T. M.: Pharmacokinetics and tolerance of ciprofloxacin after sequential increasing oral doses. Antimicrob. Agents Chemother. 29: 62-66, 1986.

Taylor, E. W., Lindsay, G., West of Scotland Surgical Infection Study Group: Antibiotic prophylaxis in transurethral resection of the prostate with reference to the influence of preoperative catheterization. J. Hosp. Infect. 12: 75-83, 1988.

Thiel, G., Spühler, O.: Katheterinfekt und sogenannte infektiöse (episomale) Resistenz. Schweiz. Med. Wschr. 95: 1155-1157, 1965.

Thompson, R. L., Haley, C. E., Searcy, M. A., Guenthner, S. M., Kaiser, D. L., Gröschel, D. H. M., Gillenwater, J. Y., Wenzel, R. P.: Catheter-associated bacteriuria. Failure to reduce attack rates using periodic instillations of a disinfectant into urinary drainage systems. JAMA 251: 747-751, 1984.

Thornton G. F., Andriole V. T.: Bacteriuria during indwelling catheter drainage. II. Effect of a closed sterile drainage system. JAMA 214: 339-342, 1970

Tilney, N. L., Strom, T. B., Vineyard, G. C., Merrill, J. P.: Factors contributing to the declining mortality rate in renal transplantation. N. Engl. J. Med. 299: 1321-1325, 1978.

Tönnesen, H., Schütten, B. T., Tollund, L., Hasselqvist, P., Klintorp, S.: Influence of alcoholism on morbidity after transurethral prostatectomy. Scand. J. Urol. Nephrol. 22: 175-177, 1988.

Trilla, A., Gatell, J. M., Mensa, J., Latorre, X., Almela, M., Soriano, E., Jimenez de Anta, M. T., San Miguel, J. G.: Risk factors for nosocomial bacteremia in a large Spanish teaching hospital: A case-control study. Infect. Control Hosp. Epidemiol. 12: 150-156, 1991.

Ueda, S., Matsuoka, K., Yamashita, T., Yoshitake, N., Yoshizumi, O., Noguchi, M., Hayashi, K., Noda, S., Eto, K.: Antibiotic prophylaxis with ofloxacin in patients undergoing transurethral prostatectomy. In: Proceedings 3rd International Symposium on New Quinolones, Vancouver, Canada, July 12-14, 1990. Eur. J. Clin. Microbiol. Infect. Dis.,(special issue): 322-323, 1991.

Vincenti, F., Amend, W. J. Jr., Feduska, N. J., Salvatierra, O. Jr.: Septic arthritis following renal transplantation. Nephron 30: 253-256, 1982.

Walker, L., King, I., Abel, B. J., Hutchison, A. G., Lewi, H. J.: Bacterial culture of the anterior urethra and its relationship to post-operative bacteriuria. Urol. Res. 14: 179-182, 1986.

Walter, S., Vejlsgaard, R.: Diagnostic catheterisation and bacteriuria in women with urinary incontinence. Br. J. Urol. 50: 106-108, 1978.

Warren, J. W., Platt, R., Thomas, R. J., Rosner, B., Kass, E. H.: Antibiotic irrigation and catheter-associated urinary-tract infections. N. Engl. J. Med. 299: 570-573, 1978.

Weidekamm, E., Portmann, R., Suter, K., Partos, C., Dell, D., Lücker, P. W.: Single- and multiple-dose pharmacokinetics of fleroxacin, a trifluorinated quinolone, in humans. Antimicrob. Agents Chemother. 31: 1909-1914, 1987.

Weidner, W., Schieffer, H. G., Dalhoff, A.: Treatment of chronic bacterial prostatitis with ciprofloxacin. Results of a one-year follow-up study. Am. J. Med. 82 (suppl 4A): 280-283, 1987.

Weiner, J. P., Gibson, G., Munster, A. M.: Use of prophylactic antibiotics in surgical procedures: Peer review guidelines as a method for quality assurance. Am. J. Surg. 139: 348-351, 1980.

Wenzel, R. P., Osterman, C. A., Hunting, K. J.: Hospital-acquired infections. II. Infection rates by site, service and common procedures in a university hospital. Am. J. Epidemiol. 104: 645-651, 1976.

Williams, M., Hole, D. J., Murdoch, R. W. G., Ogden, A. C., Hargreave, T. B.: 48-Hour cephradine and post-prostatectomy bacteriuria. Br. J. Urol. 52: 311-315, 1980.

VII. Summary

The fluoroquinolones represent a new group of highly active antimicrobial agents. Their broad antimicrobial spectrum covers all aerobic Gram-negative and Gram-positive bacteria encountered in urinary tract infections. These new quinolones are all administered orally, some also intravenously and they are usually well tolerated.

Because of these properties fluoroquinolones appear ideal antimicrobials for use in Urology. In various in vitro experiments, and animal and human studies the newer quinolones were investigated for their possible therapeutic and prophylactic use in urology. Since the benefit of antimicrobial prophylaxis in urologic surgery is highly disputed this aspect was particularly emphasized.

It was shown that the in vitro activity of several fluoroquinolones is quite stable in various media such as prostatic fluid, prostatic tissue and urine and at wide ranges of pH and inoculum sizes.

In various animal studies it was shown that fluoroquinolones reach very high tissue concentrations in urethral, vaginal and prostatic secretion and in prostatic tissue, sometimes higher than simultaneous serum concentration. This is explained by the amphoteric nature of these compounds (zwitterions).

Ciprofloxacin was found to be highly effective in preventing experimental urosurgical infections in animals. Foreign body infection could be prevented by single-dose ciprofloxacin prophylaxis.

In a pharmacokinetic study of patients with impaired renal function it was found that dose reduction of ciprofloxacin is necessary only at creatinine clearances below 50 ml/min.

Excellent clinical efficacy of ciprofloxacin was proven in a study of 161 patients with complicated urinary tract infections.

It is concluded that the newer quinolones are especially suitable for use in urological infections as well as in prophylaxis.

In an extensive review of the literature including some own studies the specific aspects of antimicrobial prophylaxis in urology are discussed and recommendations for the various urologic procedures are given.

VIII. Acknowledgments

I would like to thank all who helped me in carrying out this work and especially the coauthors of the papers forming the bases of this thesis.

I am very grateful to Prof. Paul O. Madsen who introduced me to research and for many years supported me with enthusiastic advice and generosity. Most of this work was done at his laboratory at the Veterans Administration Hospital in Madison, Wisconsin, USA.

Special thanks to Prof. Georg Rutishauser, who encouraged my research. Without his support and ongoing understanding this work would not have been possible.

I owe great thanks to Pat Rhodes and Jane Knes who helped perform many of the experiments. Thanks also to Francis McMahan who helped me with the animal studies and to Cynthia Birch who helped editing the manuscript. Funding for this publication was provided by Hoffmann La Roche, Inc., Basel.

Finally, I would like to thank Annette who was always understanding and encouraging; and my parents who were always supporting.

IX. Reprints of papers I – VII

The Influence of Various Body Fluids and pH on E. Coli MIC of Quinolone Derivatives[1]

T.C. Gasser, E.H. Larsen, T. Dørflinger and P.O. Madsen
Urology Section, William S. Middleton Memorial Veterans Hospital and
Department of Surgery, University of Wisconsin School of Medicine, Madison, WI, USA

Introduction

Great efforts have been made to treat chronic bacterial prostatitis but the results have been disappointing, possibly due to poor drug penetration in the prostate (9, 10).

The minimum inhibitory concentration (MIC) is normally determined under standardized in vitro conditions with an inoculum size of 10^4 to 10^5 bacteria in a medium with a pH of 7.2 (6). In prostatitis, however, the number of bacteria may be higher; the pH of the prostate is more basic; and there may be an interaction between body fluid and antimicrobial agents (3, 8, 11). In an earlier study we found that trimethoprim was inhibited by prostatic fluid and prostatic tissue extract and that the trimethoprim MIC decreased with increased pH (7).

To improve the treatment of chronic bacterial prostatitis, it is important to determine the influence of inoculum size, pH, and different tissue extracts on MIC. We determined the MICs of six quinolones and trimethoprim at different inoculum sizes and pH values in tissue extracts and body fluids of humans and dogs.

Material and methods

The MICs of trimethoprim and six quinolone derivatives (ciprofloxacin, norfloxacin, enoxacin, amifloxacin, ofloxacin, and A-56620) were determined with routine dilution methods against six different strains of Escherichia coli. The MIC was defined as the concentration that produced a 90% inhibition of the original inoculum.

To study the effect of inoculum size on MIC, the initial inoculum of 10^9 bacteria was serially diluted 10-fold down to 10^1, and the MICs were determined at each step.

To investigate the effect of tissue and body fluids on MIC, 1 gr of either dog prostatic tissue or human prostatic tissue was homogenized in 3 ml of phosphate buffer, pH 7. The resulting supernatant, and also dog prostatic fluid and human urine, were adjusted to pH 7 with NaOH, and MICs were determined in each medium.

To investigate the influence of pH on MIC, Mueller-Hinton broth was adjusted to pH 6, 7, or 8 with either HCl or NaOH, and the MICs were determined.

Except for the study of the inoculum size effect, the inoculum size was 10^5.

Results

The effect of inoculum size on MIC is shown in figure 1. Ciprofloxacin had the lowest and trimethoprim the highest MIC at all inoculum sizes.

Increase of the inoculum size from 10^6 to 10^9 bacteria caused a 19-fold increase of the trimethoprim MIC. In contrast, the quinolones had an increased MIC only at an inoculum size of

[1] Supported in part by the U.S. Veterans Administration

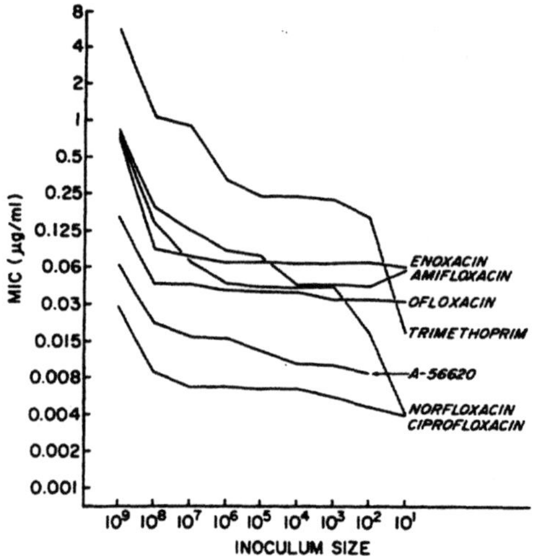

Figure 1. Effect of inoculum size on MIC of seven antimicrobials in Mueller-Hinton broth, pH 7 (means for six strains of E. coli).

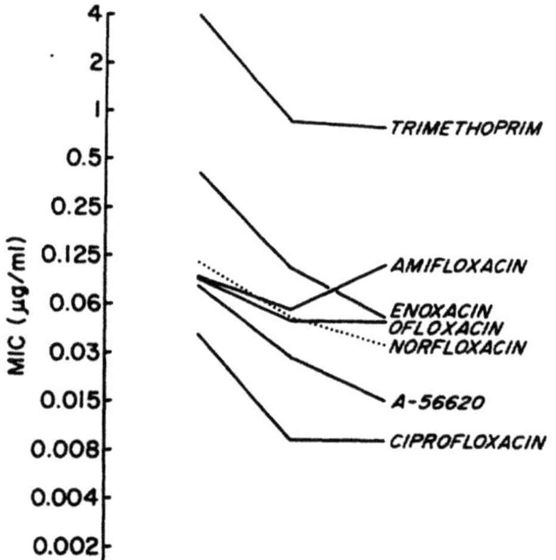

Figure 2. Effect of pH on MIC of seven antimicrobials in Mueller-Hinton broth (means for six strains of E. coli).

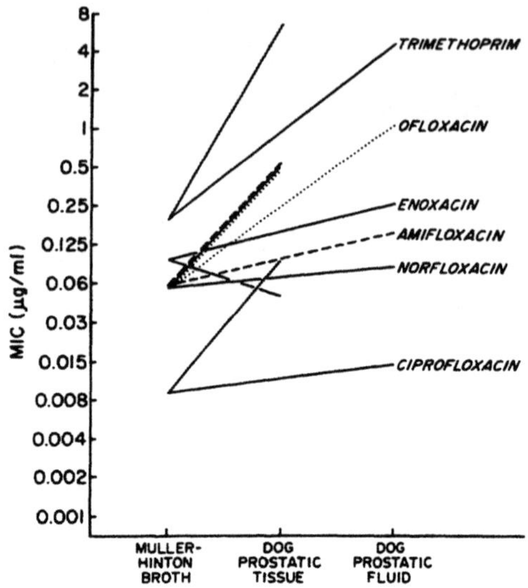

Figure 3. Influence of dog prostatic tissue and dog prostatic fluid on MIC of six antimicrobials at pH 7 (means for six strains of E. coli).

10^9, indicating that they are only slightly affected by inoculum size.

The effect of pH on MIC is shown in figure 2. Ciprofloxacin had the lowest and trimethoprim the highest MIC at each pH investigated. The MICs of all drugs decreased between pH 6 and 7. There was no MIC change between pH 7 and 8 for ciprofloxacin, ofloxacin, and trimethoprim and a slight decrease for enoxacin, norfloxacin, and A-56620. For amifloxacin, however, there was a 3.5-fold increase of MIC between pH 7 and 8.

The MICs for all drugs except enoxacin were higher in dog prostatic tissue and dog prostatic fluid (figure 3). Human prostatic tissue extract, however, had only a slight effect on the newer quinolones but clearly inhibited trimethoprim. The MIC values in human urine were higher than in Mueller-Hinton broth for all drugs investigated except for ofloxacin (figure 4).

Table I demonstrates the influence of the pH in human urine for four quinolone derivatives. The decrease of the MIC between pH 5.7 and 7 was 17-fold, 11-fold, 34-fold, and 42-fold, respectively, for enoxacin, amifloxacin, ciprofloxacin, and ofloxacin.

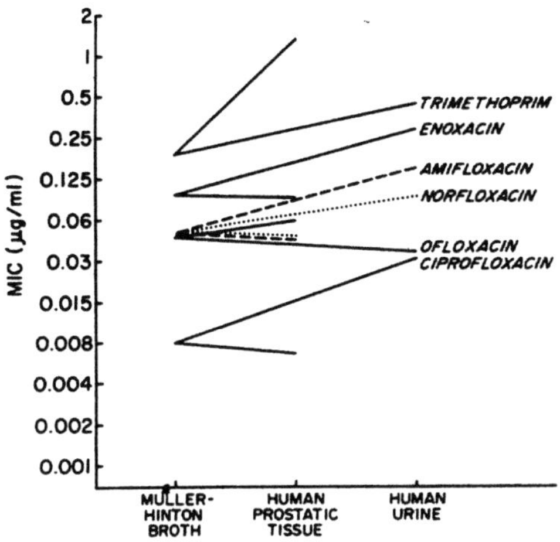

Figure 4. Influence of human prostatic tissue and human urine on MIC of six antimicrobials at pH 7 (means for six strains of E. coli).

Table I. MIC in human urine at different pH values (range for 6 strains of E. coli).

Drug	MIC, µg/ml	
	pH 5.7	pH 7
Enoxacin	5.0	0.25 -0.5
Amifloxacin	1.0 -2.0	0.125–0.25
Ciprofloxacin	0.06–2.0	0.008–0.06
Ofloxacin	1.0 -2.0	0.008–0.06

Discussion

The quinolone derivatives investigated showed an inoculum effect only at very high numbers of bacteria. This implies that they should keep their activity even if the number of bacteria is higher than under standardized in vitro conditions.

The effect of pH on MIC could be explained by changes in the degree of drug ionizaton. The ionization curves for trimethoprim, amifloxacin, and ciprofloxacin are shown in figure 5. These curves were calculated using the *Henderson-Hasselbalch* equation. Enoxacin and norfloxacin have curves similar to the one of ciprofloxacin. For a base like trimethoprim, with one pK_a, a large proportion of the drug is ionized and therefore inactive at low pH (10). Only the nonionized fraction of a drug is active, and therefore, more drug is needed to inhibit bacteria. This results in an increased MIC.

Some quinolones are zwitterions with two pK_a's. At their isoelectric point most of the drug is uncharged. At either higher or lower pH more drug is ionized and therefore inactive. Norfloxacin, enoxacin, and ciprofloxacin have the isoelectric point close to plasma pH of 7.4. At pH 6, 50 to 70% of the drug is ionized and at pH 7 only about 10% is ionized. This might explain the decrease of the MIC. At pH 8, between 15 and 30% of the drug is ionized, and one would therefore expect a slight increase of the MIC. Our results, however, show either no change or a slight decrease, possibly because high pH itself inhibits bacterial growth. The greater amount of inactive drug could be balanced by the inhibiting effect of pH 8 on bacterial growth. The isoelectric point of amifloxacin is near pH 6.6. At pH 6 and 7 the drug is 36 and 25% ionized, respectively. At pH 8, however, 70% of the drug is ionized and inactive. This may explain the MIC decrease between pH 6 and 7 and the increase between pH 7 and 8.

Therefore, in the treatment of bacterial prostatitis, where the pH is around 8 (3) one would expect better results with quinolones having either neutral or slightly basic isoelectric points (such as ciprofloxacin, norfloxacin, or enoxacin) than with quinolones having either strongly acid or basic isoelectric points.

These theoretical considerations would also explain the MIC decrease in human urine at higher pH, indicating that one should alkalinize the urine if the newer quinolones are used for the treatment of urinary tract infections.

Conclusion

Our data indicate that the pH of the medium influences the MIC of the newer quinolones, possibly because of changes in the degree of

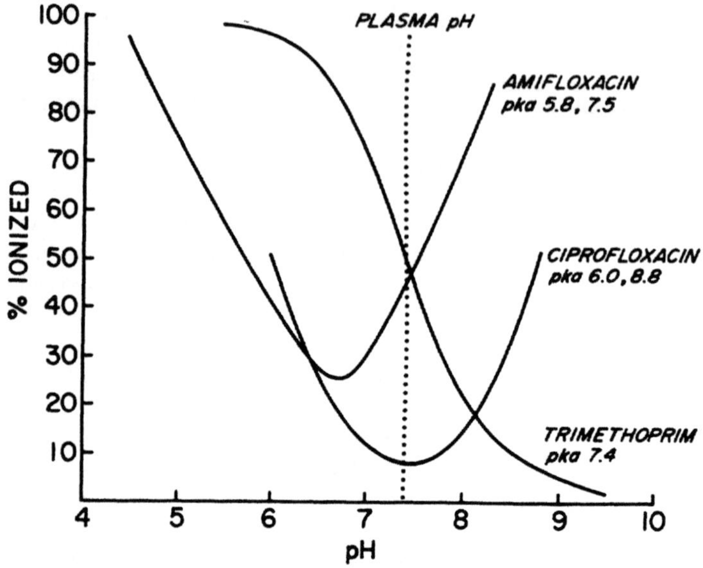

Figure 5. Ionization curves for amifloxacin, ciprofloxacin, and trimethoprim, calculated by the *Henderson-Hasselbalch* equation.

ionization of these drugs. Since the quinolones are not inhibited by human prostatic tissue extract, have a broad antibacterial spectrum, and tend to concentrate in the human prostate, we expect them to be useful drugs in the treatment of bacterial prostatitis (1, 2, 4, 5, 12).

References

1 Barry AS, Jones RN, Thornsberry C, Ayers LW, Gerlach EH, Sommers HM (1984) Antibacterial activities of ciprofloxacin, norfloxacin oxolinic acid, cinoxacin, and nalidixic acid. Antimicrob Agents Chemother 25: 633

2 Chin NX, Neu HC (1983) In vitro activity of enoxacin, a quinolone carboxylic acid, compared with those of norfloxacin, new β-lactams, aminoglycosides, and trimethoprim. Antimicrob Agents Chemother 24: 754

3 Fair WR, Cordonnier JJ (1978) The pH of prostatic fluid: a reappraisal and therapeutic implications. J Urol 120: 695

4 Iravani A, Welty GS, Newton BR, Richard GA (1985) Effects of changes in pH, medium, and inoculum size on the in vitro activity of amifloxacin against urinary isolates of Staphylococcus saprophyticus and Escherichia coli. Antimicrob Agents Chemother 27: 449

5 Jacobus NV, Tally FP, Barza M (1984) Antimicrobial sprectrum of Win 49375. Antimicrob Agents Chemother 26: 104

6 Lennette EH, Balows A, Hausler WJ Jr, Truant JP (1980) Manual of Clinical Microbiology. 3rd ed. Am Soc Microbiology, Washington, D.C., p 453

7 Madsen PO, Whalen PR (1978) Interaction between antimicrobial agents and prostatic tissue extract and fluid. Infection (suppl 1) 6: 75

8 Mett H, Gyr K, Zak O, Vosbeck K (1984) Duodeno-pancreatic secretions enhance bactericidal activity of antimicrobial drugs. Antimicrob Agents Chemother 26: 35

9 Pfau A, Sacks T (1976) Chronic bacterial prostatitis: new therapeutic aspects. Br J Urol 48: 245

10 Stamey TA, Meares EH Jr, Winningham DG (1970) Chronic bacterial prostatitis and the diffusion of drugs into prostatic fluid. J Urol 103: 187

11 Stille W (1983) The prognostic value of the antibiogram. Infection (suppl 2) 11: 66

12 Thompson DK, O'Keefe JP, Tatarowicz WA (1984) In vitro comparison of amifloxacin and six other antibiotics against aminoglycoside-resistant Pseudomonas aeruginosa. Antimicrob Agents Chemother 26: 275

Corresponding address: *Dr. P. O. Madsen*, Urology Service, William S. Middleton Memorial Veterans Hospital, 2500 Overlook Terrace, Madison, WI 53705, USA

QUINOLONE PENETRATION INTO CANINE VAGINAL AND URETHRAL SECRETIONS

T. C. Gasser, P. H. Graversen, E. H. Larsen and T. Dørflinger

From the Urology Section, William S. Middleton Memorial Veterans Hospital, Madison, Wisconsin, USA

Abstract. Four newer quinolones (amifloxacin, ciprofloxacin, enoxacin, norfloxacin) were administered to female dogs by intravenous infusion. Drug concentrations in plasma, urine, and vaginal and urethral secretion were determined by bioassay. All four quinolones penetrated into vaginal and urethral secretion in concentrations several times higher than the MIC against common urinary pathogens, ciprofloxacin and norfloxacin reaching concentrations exceeding the simultaneous plasma concentrations. Because of their favorable antibacterial spectra, new quinolones should be investigated clinically for the treatment of recurrent urinary tract infection and bacterial vaginitis.

Key words: quinolones, urinary tract infection, bacterial vaginitis.

Since the discovery of nalidixic acid and subsequent synthesis of rosoxacin and cinoxacin several years ago, the search for new antimicrobials has yielded a large number of related compounds (8). The development of 6-fluoro-7-piperazino-4-quinolones broadened and enhanced the antibacterial activity considerably. Minimal inhibitory concentrations (MIC) of the fluoroquinolones are very low against most Gram-negative bacteria, including *Pseudomonas* and Enterobacteriaceae, and they are also active against many Gram-positive organisms (1,2,5).

Colonization of the vaginal vestibule and lower urethra has been blamed for the high rate of recurrent urinary tract infections (UTIs) in women (6). Trimethoprim's popularity in the treatment and prophylaxis of UTI in women (7) has been attributed to the drug's relatively high concentration in vaginal fluid. The newer quinolones are currently being investigated as potential agents for treatment of UTIs and possibly for prophylaxis of UTI in women. As part of the investigation for the latter use, it would be helpful to know the concentrations that the drugs attain in the vaginal and urethral mucosa. If adequate concentrations are reached, new quinolones could be beneficial for treatment and prophylaxis of recurrent UTIs in women.

Results from animal studies form the basis for trials in humans. We therefore undertook drug penetration studies in dogs. Amifloxacin, ciprofloxacin, enoxacin, and norfloxacin were investigated.

MATERIAL AND METHODS

Twenty-one adult female mongrel dogs weighing between 15 and 39 kg were anaesthetized by intravenous sodium pentothal. The bladder neck was exposed through a midline abdominal incision and ligated to prevent urinary contamination of the urethral secretion. Urine was diverted through a cystostomy by a Foley catheter.

To achieve steady-state conditions, the quinolones were given intravenously as a bolus injection (10 mg/kg body weight) followed by a constant infusion of 1 mg/kg body weight for 4 hours. Pilocarpine (1 mg/kg body weight) was given i.v. at intervals as needed to stimulate vaginal and urethral secretion. Samples of vaginal secretion, urethral secretion, plasma, and urine were taken before and at 30-min intervals for 4 hours after the bolus injection. The vagina was exposed through a speculum, and two 6-mm blank paper disks (sterile blanks, Difco Laboratories, Detroit, MI) with a small thread attached for retrieval were inserted into both the urethra and the vagina. After 3-5 min in situ, they were removed and the drug concentrations of the secretion-saturated disks were determined by bioassay.

Amifloxacin disk content was determined by placing the disk direct on trypticase glucose extract agar, pH 7.0, using *Proteus vulgaris* ATC 9920 as test organism. Ciprofloxacin disk content was determined by first washing out the content in 0.2 ml phosphate buffered saline, pH 7.2. The bioassay was carried out within 24 hours in Medium C (neomycin assay agar, BBL, pH 7.2) using *Klebsiella pneumoniae* ATCC 10031 as test organism. Enoxacin disk concentration was determined by placing the disk directly on Medium 2 (Bacto Penassay Base agar, pH 7.0), using *Escherichia coli* KP as test organism. Norfloxacin disk content was determined by placing the disk directly on nutrient base yeast agar, pH 7.0, using *Klebsiella pneumoniae* ATCC 10031 as test organism.

Table I. *Concentration of quinolones in plasma, urine, and vaginal and urethral secretion*

Body fluid	Concentration of drug (μg/ml; mean ± SD)							
	30 min	60 min	90 min	120 min	150 min	180 min	210 min	240 min
	Amifloxacin (n = 5)							
Plasma	9.7±3.8	8.3±3.0	7.7±2.2	7.1±2.0	6.5±1.6	6.3±1.8	6.3±1.9	6.2±1.9
Vaginal secretion	8.9±5.3	5.7±2.8	6.1±2.7	7.0±3.8	5.9±2.4	4.4±2.5	5.3±3.5	4.9±2.4
Urethral secretion	9.3±4.8	6.9±2.8	5.9±2.8	6.9±3.9	6.1±3.1	5.8±2.9	6.2±3.8	5.4±2.9
Urine	107±121	108±137	78±104	78±111	51±81	81±144	30±32	37±57
	Ciprofloxacin (n = 5)							
Plasma	6.6±2.5	4.2±1.2	3.9±1.3	3.5±1.2	3.1±0.9	3.0±1.0	2.9±1.1	2.8±0.9
Vaginal secretion	11.6±13.5	6.8±7.4	5.4±5.4	4.9±4.9	5.3±5.7	4.3±4.0	4.4±4.0	4.4±3.8
Urethral secretion	9.5±9.8	7.4±9.9	5.3±5.1	4.5±3.6	4.5±4.1	3.9±2.9	4.1±3.2	4.4±3.5
Urine	69±118	261±214	238±157	135±60	87±57	83±32	96±64	92±75
	Enoxacin (n = 5)							
Plasma	14.3±7.0	9.7±4.6	7.1±4.1	6.1±3.9	5.3±2.7	5.4±2.5	5.1±2.4	4.9±2.2
Vaginal secretion	4.7±1.8	5.3±2.1	2.8±1.8	3.7±1.5	3.8±2.1	4.2±2.4	4.0±1.7	4.3±2.4
Urethral secretion	6.1±1.4	4.5±1.4	4.2±1.9	3.4±1.1	3.3±1.2	4.2±2.4	3.8±1.5	3.5±2.1
Urine	70±86	403±442	141±106	123±111	207±201	129±83	143±194	159±201
	Norfloxacin (n = 6)							
Plasma	5.9±1.3	5.4±1.3	4.6±0.9	3.7±0.6	3.6±0.5	3.4±0.4	3.6±0.7	3.4±0.7
Vaginal secretion	4.3±2.1	4.2±1.0	3.9±1.3	4.1±0.5	4.3±1.0	4.4±1.1	4.1±1.6	4.8±1.6
Urethral secretion	5.0±0.6	4.8±1.3	4.1±0.9	4.2±0.9	3.9±0.8	4.4±0.9	4.5±1.3	4.1±1.3
Urine	54±95	249±346	292±234	278±186	181±217	107±83	75±58	56±21

Table II. *Ratios of quinolone concentration in vaginal and urethral secretion to plasma concentration*

Type of secretion	Ratio: secretion concentration/plasma concentration (mean ± SD)							
	30 min	60 min	90 min	120 min	150 min	180 min	210 min	240 min
	Amifloxacin							
Vaginal	.96±.47	.69±.21	.76±.87	.91±.34	.90±.20	.67±.20	.76±.33	.75±.17
Urethral	.95±.30	.83±.15	.74±.16	.92±.37	.91±.30	.90±.24	.91±.31	.84±.25
	Ciprofloxacin							
Vaginal	1.43±1.50	1.43±1.32	1.27±1.19	1.27±1.19	1.67±1.83	1.44±1.40	1.56±1.49	1.82±1.35
Urethral	.84±.45	1.71±2.24	1.24±.83	1.31±1.05	1.54±1.46	1.38±1.13	1.72±1.42	1.81±1.76
	Enoxacin							
Vaginal	.51±.48	.64±.48	.61±.58	.85±.55	.80±.39	.85±.44	.75±.26	.92±.44
Urethral	.63±.54	.65±.50	.66±.32	.66±.30	.70±.23	.90±.53	.80±.24	.78±.39
	Norfloxacin							
Vaginal	.79±.45	.86±.37	.88±.31	1.14±.28	1.22±.70	1.29±.25	1.14±.30	1.40±.26
Urethral	.88±.15	.94±.36	.92±.25	1.16±.22	1.11±.26	1.29±.24	1.23±.16	1.18±.25

Plasma and urine concentrations were assayed by agar disk diffusion, using the same test media and test organisms as for the vaginal and urethral secretion.

RESULTS

The concentrations of the four quinolones investigated in plasma, urine, and vaginal and urethral secretion are shown in Table I. The concentration ratios for vaginal secretion/plasma and urethral secretion/plasma are given in Table II and are shown graphically in Fig. 1 and 2. Ciprofloxacin and norfloxacin reached ratios greater than 1.0 for both vaginal and urethral secretions, indicating that both drugs concentrate in these secretions. Amifloxacin and enoxacin also penetrated into

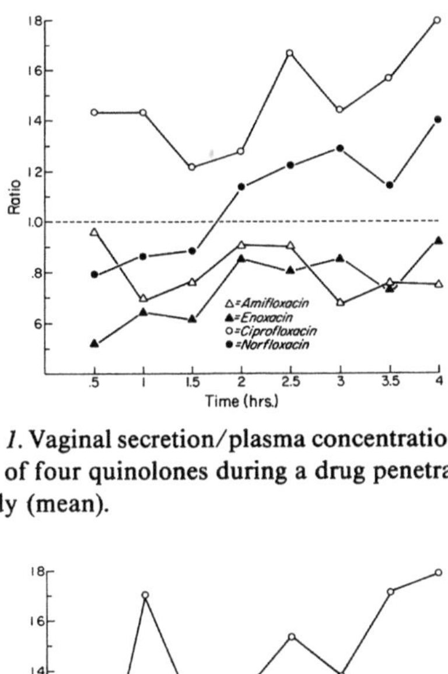

Fig. 1. Vaginal secretion/plasma concentration ratios of four quinolones during a drug penetration study (mean).

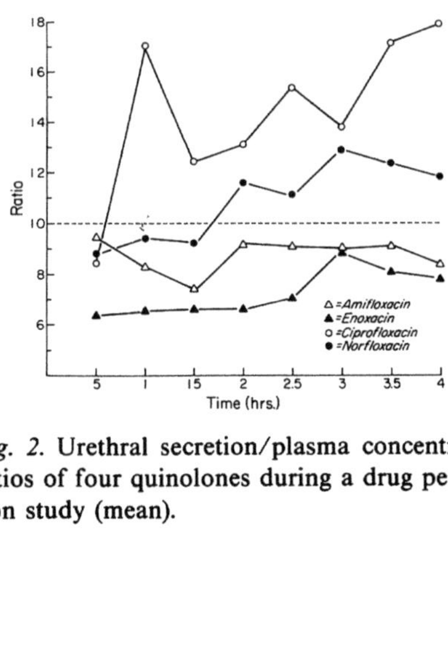

Fig. 2. Urethral secretion/plasma concentration ratios of four quinolones during a drug penetration study (mean).

vaginal and urethral secretion, but in concentrations lower than in plasma.

DISCUSSION

This study demonstrates that amifloxacin, ciprofloxacin, enoxacin, and norfloxacin penetrate into the vaginal and urethral mucosa. The mechanism of drug diffusion into the vagina is not completely clear, but is thought to be governed by the principles of passive nonionic diffusion (6,7). Only nonionized (uncharged) drug can penetrate the vaginal epithelium. The degree of ionization of a drug is determined by the drug's pKa value and the pH of the surrounding fluid. This relation is expressed in the Henderson-Hasselbalch equation:

$$\mathrm{pH} = \mathrm{pKa} + \log \frac{\text{concentration of ionized drug}}{\text{concentration of nonionized drug}}$$

At equilibrium, the highest drug concentration (charged and uncharged) is on the side of the membrane where most drug is ionized. That is, bases concentrate on the acid side and acids on the basic side. This phenomenon is called ion-trapping. Most antimicrobials are weak acids or weak bases. The quinolones investigated, however, are so-called zwitterions; i.e., they have both acidic and basic properties. Zwitterions have two ionizing groups, one positively and one negatively charged, and thus two pKa values. The ionization curves of the four drugs investigated (their degree of ionization at various pH values) are shown in Fig. 3. The Henderson-Hasselbalch equation was

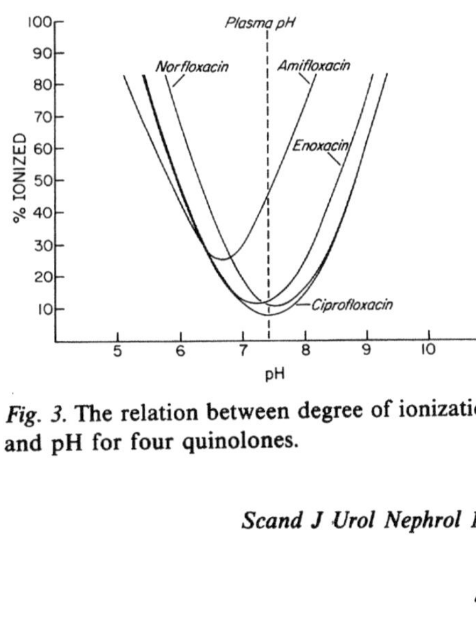

Fig. 3. The relation between degree of ionization and pH for four quinolones.

used for calculation of the curves. The minimum amount of drug is charged at the drug's isoelectric point. At higher pH values, more drug is negatively charged. Conversely, at lower pH values, more drug is positively charged.

Table III. *Theoretical concentration ratios, vaginal secretion/plasma at various pH values of vaginal secretion (plasma pH = 7.4)*

	pH		
Drug	5.0	6.0	7.0
Amifloxacin	4.1	0.9	0.8
Ciprofloxacin	10.2	1.9	1.0
Enoxacin	10.8	1.8	1.0
Norfloxacin	16.6	2.7	1.3

The theoretical vaginal secretion/plasma ratios of drug at different pH values of the vaginal secretion are listed in Table III. In dogs, plasma pH is 7.4 and the pH of vaginal and urethral secretions is 7.0 (4). In our dog experiments, good correlation was found between theoretical and actual values for amifloxacin and norfloxacin (Fig. 1). Enoxacin values were slightly lower than expected. The reason for this is not known. Other drug properties such as lipid solubility, protein binding, and molecular shape may be of influence. Actual ciprofloxacin concentration exceeded the expected values. This may be due to an active transport mechanism. However, in spite of bladder neck ligation, contamination with urine (containing high ciprofloxacin concentrations) cannot be excluded.

In humans, the pH of vaginal secretion is considerably more acid than in dogs. This would favor the penetration of the quinolones into the vagina (Table III). While the pH in uninfected women is below 4.4, it can be as high as 5.0-6.0 in infected women (6). Thus, highest concentrations in human vaginal secretion are expected for norfloxacin and lowest for amifloxacin.

Antibiotic concentrations alone, however, are not a good indicator of possible clinical efficacy. The concentration should be considered in relation to the MIC against the most common pathogens. This relation can be expressed as the inhibitory quotient or therapeutic index: drug concentration/MIC_{90} (3). The calculated therapeutic indices for the most common urinary pathogen in women, *E. coli*, are given in Table IV.

Table IV. *Therapeutic index of quinolones for E. coli*

Drug	Concentration (μg/ml) Vaginal secretion[a]	MIC_{90}[b]	Therapeutic index
Amifloxacin	5.5	0.25	22
Ciprofloxacin	5.1	0.015	340
Enoxacin	4.0	0.40	10
Norfloxacin	4.3	0.12	36

[a] Mean of 2–4 hours of drug infusion in dogs.
[b] References 1,2,5.

A therapeutic index of ≥2 is generally required for a drug to be effective. Thus all four drugs investigated are expected to be clinically effective. However, ciprofloxacin seems to be superior, mainly because of its very low MIC_{90} (1). As higher quinolone concentrations in human vaginal secretion are expected, even more favorable therapeutic indices would result for all four quinolones investigated.

The penetration properties and the favorable antimicrobial spectra of quinolones make clinical trials warranted. Determinations of quinolone concentrations in women should be followed by trials to assess the value of long-term antimicrobial prophylaxis with quinolones in women with recurrent UTI.

ACKNOWLEDGEMENT

Supported in part by the U.S. Veterans Administration.

REFERENCES

1. Barry AL, Jones RN, Thornsberry C, Ayers LW, Gerlach EH, Sommers HM. Antibacterial activities of ciprofloxacin, norfloxacin, oxolinic acid, cinoxacin, and nalidixic acid. Antimicrob Agents Chemother 1984;25:633.
2. Chin N-X, Neu HC. In vitro activity of enoxacin, a quinolone carboxylic acid, compared with those of norfloxacin, new β-lactams, aminoglycosides, and trimethoprim. Antimicrob Agents Chemother 1983;24:754.
3. Ellner PD, Neu HC. The inhibitory quotient. A method for interpreting minimal inhibitory data. JAMA 1981;246:1575.
4. Hoyme U, Baumueller A, Madsen PO. Antibiotics excretion in canine vaginal and urethral secretions. Invest Urol 1978;16:35.
5. Jacobus NV, Tally FP, Barza M. Antimicrobial spectrum of Win 49375. Antimicrob Agents Chemother 1984;26:104.
6. Stamey TA. Some observations on the pathogenesis of recurrent bacteriuria in women and children. In: Pathogenesis and Treatment of Urinary Tract Infec-

tions. Stamey TA (ed). Baltimore, Williams and Wilkins, 1980 pp 210-289.
7. Stamey TA, Condy M. The diffusion and concentration of trimethoprim in human vaginal fluid. J Infect Dis 1975;131:261.
8. Wolfson JS, Hooper DC. The fluoroquinolones: structures, mechanisms of action and resistance, and spectra of activity in vitro. Antibicrob Agents Chemother 1985;28:581.

Antimicrobial Agents and Chemotherapy, July 1987, p. 1010–1013 Vol. 31, No. 7
0066-4804/87/071010-04$02.00/0

Fleroxacin (Ro 23-6240) Distribution in Canine Prostatic Tissue and Fluids

THOMAS C. GASSER,† PEDER H. GRAVERSEN, AND PAUL O. MADSEN*

Urology Section, Surgical Service, William S. Middleton Memorial Veterans Administration Hospital, Madison, Wisconsin 53705

Received 16 January 1987/Accepted 29 April 1987

The distribution of fleroxacin (Ro 23-6240) in canine prostatic tissue and fluids was investigated under steady-state conditions during intravenous infusion. Mean ratios of fleroxacin concentration in tissue and fluids over concentration in plasma were 1.57 ± 0.25 for prostatic tissue, 1.12 ± 0.28 for prostatic secretion, and 0.93 ± 0.14 for prostatic interstitial fluid. These levels and concentrations in urine were several times higher than the MIC for most pathogens that cause chronic bacterial prostatitis and urinary tract infection. The MICs for several isolates of *Escherichia coli* were only slightly affected by canine prostatic secretion, human prostatic tissue extract, and human urine. Clinical trials with fleroxacin appear justified for chronic bacterial prostatitis and urinary tract infection.

Chronic bacterial prostatitis may be the most common cause of recurrent urinary tract infection in men (20). Despite the availability of antimicrobial agents with suitable antibacterial spectra, results of treating chronic bacterial prostatitis have been rather disappointing. The best cure rates reported, using trimethoprim-sulfamethoxazole for 4 to 16 weeks, vary from 32 to 71% (19).

Fleroxacin (Ro 23-6240 or AM-833) is a newly developed quinolone derivative structurally related to the latest generation of 6-fluoro-7-piperazine-4-quinolones. It has a broad antibacterial spectrum against both gram-positive and gram-negative bacteria, including *Pseudomonas aeruginosa* and the *Enterobacteriaceae* (4, 8, 10). Fleroxacin is well absorbed after oral administration in experimental animals (13), and its long half-life of 9 to 11 h may allow once-per-day dosing (data on file, Hoffmann-La Roche, Inc.). Its antibacterial and pharmacokinetic properties make fleroxacin a potential drug for the treatment of urologic infections, possibly including chronic bacterial prostatitis.

The purpose of this study was to evaluate the distribution of fleroxacin in plasma, prostatic secretion, prostatic interstitial fluid, prostatic tissue, and urine of dogs. We investigated in vitro the influence of dog prostatic secretion, human prostatic tissue extract, and human urine on the antibacterial activity of fleroxacin.

MATERIALS AND METHODS

Animal studies. Fleroxacin was obtained from Hoffmann-La Roche, Inc., Nutley, N.J. The dog model used for drug infusion studies has been previously described (15). Five adult male mongrel dogs weighing 23 to 33 kg were anesthetized intravenously with sodium thiopental. The prostrate was exposed through a low midline abdominal incision, and a multiperforated polyethylene tissue chamber (10 by 6 mm) with two connecting tubes (Engineering Industries, Verona, Wis.) was implanted in each lateral lobe (Fig. 1). The tubes were irrigated with heparin and placed subcutaneously. Approximately 4 weeks later, the dogs were anesthetized again. The bladder neck was ligated, and a vasectomy was performed to prevent contamination of the prostatic secretion. Prostatic secretion was collected through a transurethrally inserted catheter; prostatic interstitial fluid was obtained from the tissue chambers via the tubes. Urine was collected through a cystostomy. Blood samples were drawn through a cannula inserted in the femoral artery.

To achieve steady-state conditions, fleroxacin was given intravenously as a bolus injection (10 mg/kg of body weight) followed by constant infusion of 1 mg/kg of body weight for 4 h. The infusion rate was doubled in three of the dogs after 3 h and extended to 5 h. To stimulate prostatic secretion, pilocarpine (0.1 mg/kg of body weight) was administered intravenously at intervals as needed. Samples of plasma, urine, prostatic interstitial fluid, and prostatic secretion were collected before drug administration and subsequently at 30-min intervals until the end of the experiment. The dogs were then sacrificed, and specimens from various tissues were taken for bioassay.

All samples were frozen immediately and stored at −17°C until used for bioassay. Fleroxacin concentrations were determined by bioassay, using a disk diffusion method. The test medium was tryptose glucose agar (pH 7.2; GIBCO Diagnostics, Madison, Wis.), and the test organism was *Bacillus subtillis* ATCC 6633 (Difco Laboratories, Detroit, Mich.). Tissue samples were weighed and then homogenized with an equal volume of phosphate buffer (pH 7.2) by using a Polytron 10 homogenizer (Kinematica GmbH, Luzern, Switzerland), and the supernatant was removed. Urine samples were diluted 1:25 in phosphate buffer (pH 7.2). Plasma, prostatic secretion, and prostatic interstitial fluid were not diluted. Standard curves for plasma were generated from pooled normal dog plasma. A phosphate buffer (pH 7.2) was used for standard curves for prostatic secretion, prostatic interstitial fluid, tissues, and urine. All samples were assayed in triplicate and incubated at 37°C overnight before inhibition zones were measured.

To study the effect of body fluids on the antibacterial activity of fleroxacin, samples of canine prostatic secretion, human prostatic tissue (obtained from patients with benign prostatic hyperplasia, undergoing transurethral resection of the prostate), and human urine were collected. The extract of human prostatic tissue was obtained by homogenizing prostatic tissue with an equal volume of phosphate buffer

* Corresponding author.
† Present address: Urology Section, University Hospital, 4031 Basel, Switzerland.

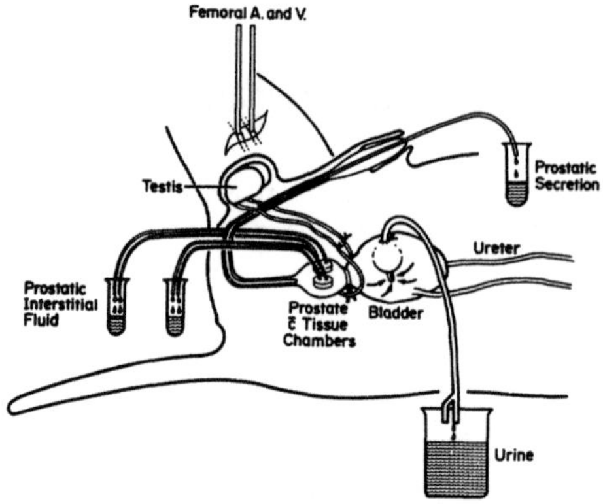

FIG. 1. Dog model with implanted tissue chambers in the prostate.

(pH 7.2) and removing the supernatant. MIC determinations were performed at existing pH levels of fluids and extracts, and all samples were then adjusted to pH 7.0 with 0.1 N sodium hydroxide. The MIC was determined by using a twofold dilution technique with Mueller-Hinton broth plus body fluids and extracts. The final dilutions, containing 10^5 *Escherichia coli* per ml (obtained from 12 different patients with urinary tract infection), were incubated overnight at 37°C with the antibacterial agent. At the end of this period, the MIC was defined as the concentration in the last clear well.

For statistical calculations, we employed Student's *t* test and the Mann-Whitney rank-sum test; *P* values of <0.05 were considered significant.

RESULTS

All tissue chambers yielded sufficient amounts of fluid every 30 min for bioassay. The prostatic interstitial fluid values are averages for the two chambers. Table 1 shows mean values of fleroxacin concentrations in plasma, prostatic secretion, prostatic interstitial fluid, and urine along with the prostatic secretion/plasma and prostatic interstitial fluid/plasma concentration ratios. Assuming that a steady state had occurred after 1.5 h, the mean concentrations were significantly higher in prostatic secretion than in prostatic interstitial fluid ($P < 0.001$); the prostatic secretion/plasma concentration ratios were constantly above 1. Some dogs had relatively small urine output in the beginning of the study period, which may explain the high urine concentrations recorded from 0.5 to 1.5 h.

TABLE 2. Concentrations and tissue/plasma concentration ratios of fleroxacin in various tissues at autopsy[a]

Tissue	Concn (µg/g)	Tissue/plasma ratio
Prostate	11.0 ± 2.6	1.57 ± 0.25
Testis	11.4 ± 2.3	1.67 ± 0.35
Epididymis	11.1 ± 4.3	1.56 ± 0.40
Bladder wall	11.1 ± 3.9	1.63 ± 0.37
Kidney cortex	19.8 ± 6.5	2.91 ± 1.23
Kidney medulla	20.4 ± 5.8	3.04 ± 0.80

[a] Mean ± standard deviation.

Various lower genitourinary tissue concentrations and corresponding tissue/plasma concentration ratios are shown in Table 2. Table 3 shows the influence of various body fluids in the MIC of fleroxacin. Canine prostatic secretion, human prostatic tissue extract, and human urine had only a slight effect; the MICs for 90% of isolates tested at pH 7.0 in human prostatic tissue extract and human urine did not differ significantly from the values obtained in Mueller-Hinton broth (results not shown). Conversely, lowering the pH values in the medium increased the MICs significantly ($P < 0.01$).

DISCUSSION

This study demonstrated that fleroxacin penetrates well into lower genitourinary tissues and secretions of dogs. The concentrations of fleroxacin in prostatic secretion, prostatic interstitial fluid, and urine were many times higher than the MIC for most urinary tract pathogens (4, 10, 18).

To treat chronic bacterial prostatitis successfully, adequate drug levels must be achieved in the prostate. Penetration into the prostate is thought to be a passive process and depends on many physicochemical properties, such as degree of ionization, protein binding, and lipid solubility (22). In this study, prostatic secretion/plasma and prostatic interstitial fluid/plasma concentration ratios close to 1 were not changed by increasing the plasma concentration of fleroxacin (Table 1). This suggests that the drug is passively diffused from plasma into the prostate and is in accordance with the theory proposed by Stamey et al. (22). The ideal drug is uncharged at plasma pH, has low protein binding, and is lipophilic. In addition to these factors, the presence of a pH gradient across the prostatic epithelium is also important because of the phenomenon of ion trapping. When steady-state conditions have occurred, the highest drug concentration will be on the side of the biological membrane where most ionization occurs (i.e., charged plus uncharged). This is dependent on the pK_a of the drug and the pH of the medium. This relation is expressed by the Henderson-Hasselbalch equation (22). Whereas most antimicrobial drugs are either weak acids or bases (with 1 pK_a), newer

TABLE 1. Concentration of fleroxacin in fluids in five dogs

Fluid[a]	Concn (µg/ml; mean ± SD) at time[b]:									
	0.5 h	1.0 h	1.5 h	2.0 h	2.5 h	3.0 h	3.5 h	4.0 h	4.5 h	5.0 h
P	7.6 ± 1.0	7.0 ± 0.6	6.6 ± 0.8	6.5 ± 1.0	6.3 ± 0.7	6.2 ± 0.9	6.9 ± 1.0	6.8 ± 1.5	7.6 ± 2.1	8.1 ± 1.9
PS	13.5 ± 1.6	9.2 ± 1.4	7.2 ± 1.6	7.2 ± 1.4	6.9 ± 1.6	6.5 ± 1.5	7.2 ± 1.8	7.2 ± 1.6	9.4 ± 2.3	9.4 ± 1.8
PIF	9.2 ± 3.8	8.4 ± 3.6	6.6 ± 1.5	5.8 ± 1.4	5.9 ± 1.8	5.7 ± 1.7	5.7 ± 1.8	6.3 ± 1.7	7.7 ± 2.1	8.2 ± 1.9
Urine	149 ± 226	176 ± 141	154 ± 152	94 ± 50	104 ± 98	124 ± 129	66 ± 29	67 ± 48	76 ± 24	63 ± 38
PS/P	1.80 ± 0.25	1.34 ± 0.35	1.12 ± 0.38	1.13 ± 0.37	1.12 ± 0.28	1.06 ± 0.31	1.05 ± 0.23	1.07 ± 0.22	1.26 ± 0.26	1.16 ± 0.16
PIF/P	1.10 ± 0.26	1.20 ± 0.32	0.99 ± 0.20	0.88 ± 0.20	0.94 ± 0.19	0.91 ± 0.18	0.80 ± 0.16	0.91 ± 0.10	1.00 ± 0.05	1.00 ± 0.07

[a] P, Plasma; PS, prostatic secretion; PIF, prostatic interstitial fluid.
[b] Between 3.5 and 5 h, data from only three dogs were compiled.

TABLE 3. Effect of various body fluids on the MIC of fleroxacin for 12 isolates of *Escherichia coli*

Body fluid	pH	MIC (μg/ml)[a]		
		Range	50%	90%
Dog prostatic secretion	6.5	1.0–1.0	1.0	1.0
Dog prostatic secretion	7.0	0.03–1.0	0.06	0.125
Human prostatic tissue extract	7.0	0.06–1.0	0.125	0.25
Human urine	5.0	0.25–>1.0	1.0	1.0
Human urine	7.0	0.06–0.5	0.125	0.25

[a] 50% and 90%, MIC for 50 and 90% of isolates, respectively.

quinolone drugs have two ionizing groups, one positively and the other negatively charged, and thus two pK_as (the so-called zwitterions, or dipolar ions). The two pK_as of fleroxacin are 5.5 and 8.1. Figure 2 shows the calculated ionization curve for fleroxacin. As only the uncharged fraction is diffusible and active (22), the lowest MIC is expected at the drug's isoelectric point. At both higher and lower pH values more drug is charged, resulting in an increased MIC. This pH effect was demonstrable in canine prostatic secretion and human urine (Table 3) and suggests that it might be worthwhile to adjust pH to around 7.0 when treating urinary tract infections with fleroxacin.

Interaction between body fluids and antimicrobial agents has been previously described (16, 21). In our study, however, the investigated body fluids had no significant effect on MIC, indicating that the antibacterial activity of fleroxacin would be unaffected by prostatic secretion and urine.

The prostatic secretion/plasma ratio of fleroxacin (Fig. 3) was compared with ratios found for six other quinolones studied in our laboratory, using the same dog model (6, 8, 9, 12, 17). Only fleroxacin and enoxacin had prostatic secretion/plasma concentration ratios constantly above 1. Although the results obtained from canine studies cannot be extrapolated to humans without caution, we would expect to find high prostatic concentrations of fleroxacin in humans. In humans, the pH of prostatic secretions is neutral or slightly alkaline, and in men with prostatitis, the pH may be as high as 8.3 (7). Theoretically, this should favor the penetration of most of the quinolones into the prostate. Published data on clinical studies with the quinolones and the prostate are

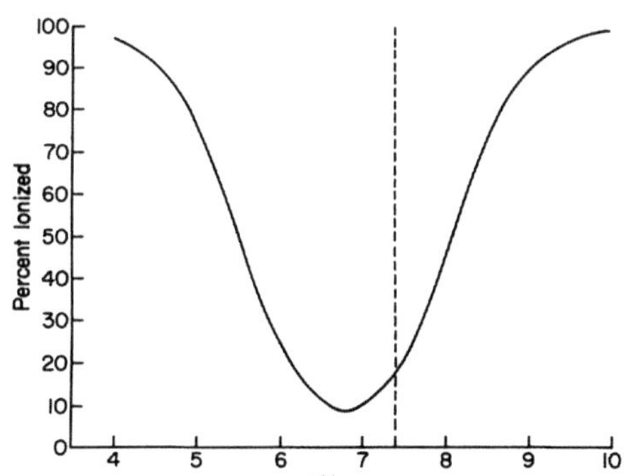

FIG. 2. Ionization curve for fleroxacin, using the Henderson-Hasselbalch equation for calculation.

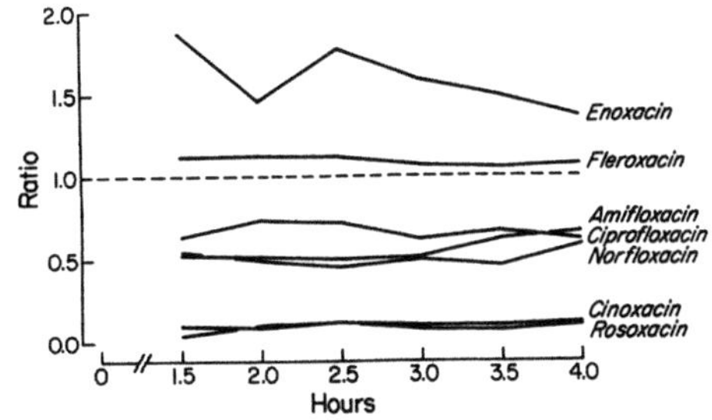

FIG. 3. Prostatic secretion/plasma concentration ratios of fleroxacin compared with those of six other quinolones.

currently limited to determination of concentrations in prostatic tissue and fluids. Several quinolones (i.e., norfloxacin, enoxacin, and ciprofloxacin) have been shown to concentrate in human prostatic tissue in concentrations substantially above the MIC for most urinary tract pathogens (1–3, 5, 11, 14).

Our findings, along with the favorable broad antimicrobial activity of fleroxacin, indicate that it might be a promising new drug for the treatment of urologic infections, including bacterial prostatitis.

ACKNOWLEDGMENT

This work was supported in part by the Veterans Administration.

LITERATURE CITED

1. **Bergeron, M. G., M. Thabet, R. Roy, C. Lessard, and P. Foucault.** 1985. Norfloxacin penetration into human renal and prostatic tissues. Antimicrob. Agents Chemother. **28**:349–350.
2. **Boerema, J. B. J., A. Dalhoff, and F. M. Y. Debruyne.** 1985. Ciprofloxacin distribution in prostatic tissue and fluid following oral administration. Chemotherapy **31**:13–18.
3. **Bologna, M., L. Vaggi, C. M. Forchetti, and E. Martini.** 1983. Bactericidal intraprostatic concentrations of norfloxacin. Lancet, **ii**:280.
4. **Chin, N.-X., D. C. Brittain, and H. C. Neu.** 1986. In vitro activity of Ro 23-6240, a new fluorinated 4-quinolone. Antimicrob. Agents Chemother. **29**:675–680.
5. **Dalhoff, A., and W. Weidner.** 1984. Diffusion of ciprofloxacin into prostatic fluid. Eur. J. Clin. Microbiol. **3**:360–362.
6. **Dørflinger, T., and P. O. Madsen.** 1985. Enoxacin concentrations in prostatic tissue, prostatic secretion, interstitial fluid, and other tissues: an experimental study in dogs. J. Int. Biomed. Info. Data **6**:41–44.
7. **Fair, W. R., and J. J. Cordonnier.** 1978. The pH of prostatic fluid: a reappraisal and therapeutic implications. J. Urol. **120**:695–698.
8. **Frimodt-Møller, P. C., T. Dørflinger, and P. O. Madsen.** 1984. Distribution of ciprofloxacin in the dog prostate and various tissues. Urol. Res. **12**:283–286.
9. **Frimodt-Møller, P. C., T. Dørflinger, and P. O. Madsen.** 1985. Amifloxacin distribution in the dog prostate. Prostate **6**:163–168.
10. **Hirai, K., H. Aoyama, M. Hosaka, Y. Oomori, Y. Niwata, S. Suzue, and T. Irikura.** 1986. In vitro and in vivo antibacterial activity of AM-833, a new quinolone derivative. Antimicrob. Agents Chemother. **29**:1059–1066.
11. **Hoogkamp-Korstanje, J. A. A., H. J. van Oort, J. J. Schipper, and T. van der Wal.** 1984. Intraprostatic concentration of ciprofloxacin and its activity against urinary pathogens. J. Antimicrob. Chemother. **14**:641–645.
12. **Jensen, K. M.-E., and P. O. Madsen.** 1983. Distribution of quinolone carboxylic acid derivatives in the dog prostate. Pros-

tate **4**:407–414.

13. **Kusajima, H., N. Ishikawa, M. Machida, H. Uchida, and T. Irikura.** 1986. Pharmacokinetics of a new quinolone, AM-833, in mice, rats, rabbits, dogs, and monkeys. Antimicrob. Agents Chemother. **30**:304–309.
14. **Larsen, E. H., T. C. Gasser, T. Dørflinger, and P. O. Madsen.** 1986. The concentration of various quinolone derivatives in the human prostate, p. 40–44. *In* W. Weidner (ed.), Therapy of prostatitis. W. Zuckwerdt Verlag, Munich.
15. **Madsen, P. O., A. Baumueller, and U. Hoyme.** 1978. Experimental models for determination of antimicrobials in prostatic tissue, interstitial fluid and secretion. Scand. J. Infect. Dis. Suppl. **14**:145–150.
16. **Madsen, P. O., and P. R. Whalen.** 1978. Interaction between antimicrobial agents and prostatic tissue extract and fluid. Infection **6**:S75–S77.
17. **Maigaard, S., N. Frimodt-Møller, U. Hoyme, and P. O. Madsen.** 1979. Rosoxacin and cinoxacin distribution in prostate, vagina, and female urethra. Invest. Urol. **17**:149–152.
18. **Manek, N., J. M. Andrews, and R. Wise.** 1986. In vitro activity of Ro 23-6240, a new difluoroquinolone derivative, compared with that of other antimicrobial agents. Antimicrob. Agents Chemother. **30**:330–332.
19. **Meares, E. M., Jr.** 1980. Prostatitis syndromes: new perspectives about old woes. J. Urol. **123**:141–147.
20. **Meares, E. M., Jr., and T. A. Stamey.** 1968. Bacteriologic localization patterns in bacterial prostatitis and urethritis. Invest. Urol. **5**:492–518.
21. **Mett, H., K. Gyr, O. Zak, and K. Vosbeck.** 1984. Duodenopancreatic secretions enhance bactericidal activity of antimicrobial drugs. Antimicrob. Agents Chemother. **26**:35–38.
22. **Stamey, T. A., E. M. Meares, Jr., and D. G. Winningham.** 1970. Chronic bacterial prostatitis and the diffusion of drugs into prostatic fluid. J. Urol. **103**:187–194.

FAC Fortschritte der antimikrobiellen u. antineoplastischen Chemotherapie Band 6–10, 1987 S. 2027-2032
ISSN 0722-7566 ISBN 3-923599-34-X

Vergleichende Pharmakokinetik in der Prostata*

T. C. GASSER, P. H. GRAVERSEN, E. H. LARSEN, P. O. MADSEN

William S. Middleton Memorial Veterans Hospital, Urology Section, Madison, Wisconsin 53705, U.S.A.

Einleitung

Die chronisch bakterielle Prostatitis ist ein schwer zu behandelndes Krankheitsbild. Die besten Heilungsraten von nur 32–71% bei Langzeitbehandlung mit Trimethoprim-Sulfamethoxazol (9) werden mit schlechter Diffusion des Medikaments in die Prostata erklärt (10).

Neuere Chinolone besitzen ein antibakterielles Spektrum, das die meisten der Prostatitis verursachenden Bakterien beinhaltet (1, 4, 6); sie könnten deshalb von Nutzen in der Behandlung der chronisch bakteriellen Prostatitis sein. Um Einblick in die Pharmakokinetik dieser neuen antibakteriellen Substanzen zu gewinnen, haben wir in unserem Tierlabor die Diffusion von sieben Chinolonen in die Hundeprostata unter Steady-state-Bedingungen untersucht. Das verwendete Tiermodell wurde bereits von *Madsen* et al. beschrieben (8).

Material und Methoden

Ausgewachsenen Hunden (Gewicht: 15–35 kg) wurden in Narkose zwei 10 × 6 mm große perforierte Gewebekammern in die Prostata implantiert (Abb. 1). Bei zu kleiner Prostata wurde nur eine Kammer eingebracht. Die Kanülen der Kammern wurden nach Spülung mit Heparin subkutan plaziert.

Einen Monat später wurden die Hunde erneut anästhesiert und der Blasenhals sowie die Vasa deferentia ligiert. Prostatasekret (PS) wurde mittels transurethralem Katheter, interstitielle Prostataflüssigkeit (IPF) durch die Gewebekammern und Plasma (P) mittels Arteria-femoralis-Katheter gewonnen.

Nach einer i.v. Bolusinjektion von 10 mg/kg Körpergewicht (KG) wurden die Chinolone mit 1–3 mg/kg KG/Stunde für vier Stunden i.v. infundiert.

Die Prostatasekretion wurde mit Pilocarpin (0,1 mg/kg KG) stimuliert. Proben von P, PS und IPF wurden vor und in 30minütigen Intervallen nach Beginn der Infusion gewonnen.

Am Ende des Experiments wurden die Hunde getötet und Gewebeproben zur Bestimmung der Chinolonkonzentration aus der Prostata entnommen. Alle Proben wurden bis zur Weiterverarbeitung bei −17° C aufbewahrt.

Die Cinoxacinkonzentration wurde mittels Fluorometrie, die Konzentrationen der übrigen sechs Chinolone mittels Bioassay bestimmt.

* *Unterstützt durch die Veterans Administration der U.S.A.*

***Keywords:** Prostatitis – Trimethoprim-Sulfamethoxazol – Pharmakokinetik – Tiermodell Hundeprostata – Chinolone – Prostatasekretion*

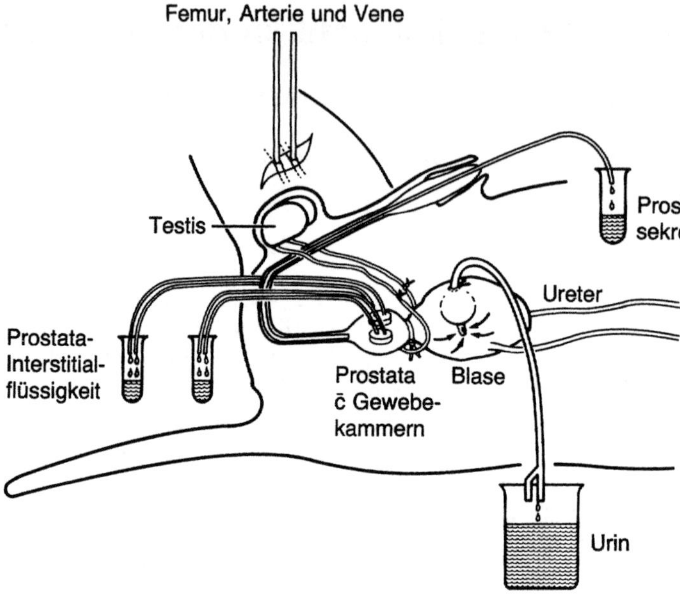

Abbildung 1: Schematische Zeichnung des verwendeten Hundemodells mit in die Prostata implantierten Gewebekammern

Tabelle 1: Konzentration von sieben Chinolonen in Plasma und Prostata des Hundes (μg/ml, Mittel und Streuung) während konstanter Infusion

Chinolon	Plasma	Prostatasekret	Interstitielle Prostataflüssigkeit	Prostatagewebe (μg/g)
Enoxacin	2,9 (2,3– 3,2)	4,2 (1,9– 5,5)	3,6 (2,3– 4,5)	5,8 (2,6–12,0)
A-56620	5,4 (3,1– 7,7)	6,6 (3,8– 9,0)	5,6 (2,5– 9,5)	5,8 (1,7– 7,2)
Ciprofloxacin	6,0 (3,6– 9,9)	3,4 (1,8– 7,5)	3,2 (1,6– 5,4)	4,0 (3,1– 4,7)
Norfloxacin	3,8 (2,7–11,1)	2,1 (0,7– 5,1)	2,3 (1,5– 4,5)	3,2 (2,0– 5,7)
Amifloxacin	12,0 (9,0–19,0)	6,3 (3,6–15,0)	6,7 (4,2–20,0)	9,4 (5,8–11,2)
Rosoxacin	11,1 (6,0–18,0)	1,1 (0,4– 2,0)	2,9 (1,5– 4,5)	3,7 (2,8– 5,2)
Cinoxacin	45 (37 –52)	1,0 (0,5– 2,6)	5,0 (2,4–29,6)	2,8 (2,3– 5,1)

Ergebnisse

Die Konzentrationen der sieben untersuchten Chinolone in P, PS und IPF sind in Tabelle 1 aufgeführt. Das Erreichen des Steady-state-Zustandes wurde nach 120 min angenommen. In Abbildung 2 ist ein graphischer Vergleich der PS/P-Quotienten der sieben Chinolone dargestellt. Alle untersuchten Chinolone konnten im PS nachgewiesen werden, aber nur Enoxacin und A-56620 erreich-

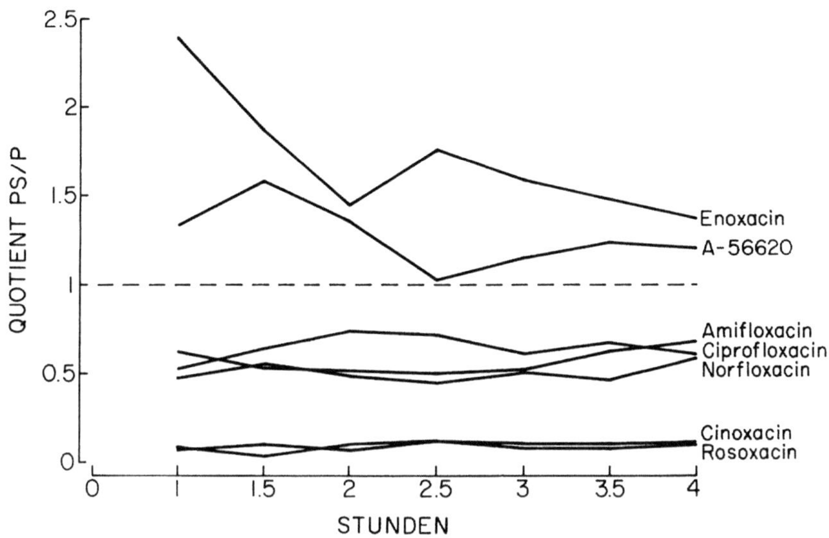

Abbildung 2: Prostatasekretion (PS)/Plasma (P)-Konzentrationsquotienten von sieben Chinolonen während einer Infusionsstudie beim Hund

ten Quotienten größer als 1,0 (d. h. sie konzentrierten im PS). Ähnliche Verhältnisse wurden auch in IPF und Prostatagewebe gefunden (Tab. 1).

Diskussion

In den 60er Jahren führte *Stamey* Diffusionsstudien antibakterieller Substanzen im Hundemodell durch, um Verständnis für das häufige Versagen antibakterieller Therapie bei Patienten mit chronisch bakterieller Prostatitis zu gewinnen (10). Während die basischen Substanzen Erythromycin und Oleandomycin im PS in höheren Konzentrationen als im Plasma gefunden wurden, konnten trotz hoher Plasmaspiegel keine der sauren Medikamente nachgewiesen werden. Aufgrund dieser Beobachtung wandte *Stamey* die Theorie der passiven, nichtionischen Diffusion auf die Prostata an. Diese besagt, daß nur ungeladene (= nichtionisierte) Partikel eine biologische Membran passieren können. Der Ionisierungsgrad einer Substanz ist abhängig von ihrem pK_a und dem pH des umgebenden Mediums, ausgedrückt durch die *Henderson-Hasselbalch*-Gleichung:

$$pH = pK_a + \log [A^-]/[AH]$$

Im Gleichgewichtszustand findet sich die höhere Gesamtkonzentration (geladen und ungeladen) der Substanz auf der Seite des höheren Ionisierungsgrades.

Bei einem pH im Plasma von 7,4 ist praktisch 100% der Säure Cinoxacin (pK_a 4,7) negativ ionisiert und somit unfähig, in die Hundeprostata (pH 6,4) zu penetrieren (Abb. 3). Der erwartet tiefe PS/P-Quotient wurde experimentell bestätigt. Rosoxacin (pK_a 8,5) ist ebenfalls eine Säure und sollte nicht im PS konzentrieren. Der gefundene Wert – deut-

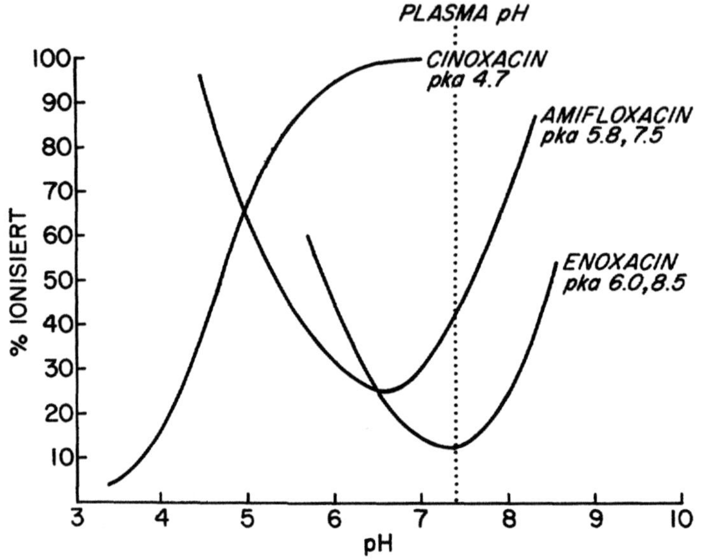

Abbildung 3: Ionisationskurven von Cinoxacin, Amifloxacin und Enoxacin, berechnet mit der *HENDERSON-HASSELBALCH*-Gleichung

lich tiefer als erwartet – ist möglicherweise mit der hohen Eiweißbindung der Substanz zu erklären (11).

Enoxacin, Ciprofloxacin, Amifloxacin und Norfloxacin sind weder Säuren noch Basen, sondern besitzen beide Eigenschaften (= Zwitterionen) und haben deshalb U-förmige Ionisationskurven (Abb. 3). Am isoelektrischen Punkt ist ein Minimum an Substanz ionisiert. Amifloxacin (pK_{a1} 5,8; pK_{a2} 7,5) mit dem isoelektrischen Punkt nahe dem pH des PS sollte auf der Plasmaseite (höherer Ionisationsgrad bei pH 7,4) konzentrieren, während Enoxacin (pK_{a1} 6,0; pK_{a2} 8,5) mit dem isoelektrischen Punkt nahe dem pH des Plasmas im PS in höherer Konzentration gefunden werden sollte. Ciprofloxacin (pK_{a1} 6,0; pK_{a2} 8,8) und Norfloxacin (pK_{a1} 6,3; pK_{a2} 8,8) haben sehr ähnliche isoelektrische Punkte (und Ionisationskurven) wie Enoxacin und sollten ebenfalls im PS konzentrieren.

Die Gründe dafür, warum erwarteter und tatsächlicher Wert nur bei Amifloxacin und Enoxacin übereinstimmen, nicht aber bei Ciprofloxacin und Norfloxacin, sind nicht bekannt. Andere Substanzeigenschaften wie Eiweißbindung, Fettlöslichkeit oder stochastische Eigenheiten könnten eine Rolle spielen. Ihr Einfluß ist jedoch schwierig zu untersuchen. Es ist unklar, weshalb A-56620 (3 pK_a's!) in der Hundeprostata konzentriert.

Da der pH-Wert des menschlichen PS neutral oder leicht alkalisch ist (5), existiert praktisch kein pH-Gefälle zwischen PS und P, und für die neueren Chinolone ist ein Quotient nahe 1 zu erwarten. Da jedoch deutlich höhere Prostatagewebe/Plasma-Quotienten für Norfloxacin, Ciprofloxacin und Enoxacin gefunden wurden (Tab. 2) (2, 3, 7), muß ein spezifischer aktiver Transportmechanismus für diese fluorierten Chinolone in die menschliche Prostata vermutet werden. Die Annahme eines solchen aktiven Transportmechanismus ist spekulativ, wird

Tabelle 2: Konzentration von Norfloxacin, Ciprofloxacin und Enoxacin in Plasma und Prostata des Menschen (Mittel und Standardabweichung) (5)

Chinolon	Plasma (P) (µg/ml)	Prostatagewebe (G) (µg/g)	Quotient (P/G)
Norfloxacin	1,2 ± 0,6	2,2 ± 0,8	1,86 ± 0,47
Ciprofloxacin	1,7 ± 1,0	3,2 ± 2,8	2,05 ± 1,46
Enoxacin	2,1 ± 0,6	4,9 ± 1,7	2,48 ± 1,17

aber unterstützt durch die Tatsache, daß die gefundenen Prostatagewebekonzentrationen sowohl beim Hund wie beim Menschen in derselben Größenordnung liegen (Tab. 1 und 2), obwohl im Hundeplasma höhere Plasmawerte vorlagen als beim Menschen. Bei rein passiver Diffusion würde man eine direkte Proportionalität zwischen Plasma- und Gewebekonzentration erwarten.

Wenn auch die theoretische Basis für die gefundenen Konzentrationen nicht ganz klar ist, so könnte diese doch klinisch bedeutsam sein. Die Konzentrationen von Enoxacin, Norfloxacin und Ciprofloxacin in Plasma und Prostatagewebe des Menschen sind deutlich höher als die minimale Hemmkonzentration (MHK) der meisten pathogenen Organismen, einschließlich so problematischer Keime wie Pseudomonas, Klebsiella oder Enterobacter spp. (12). Für E. coli, einem häufigen Verursacher der chronisch bakteriellen Prostatitis (10), liegen die Konzentrationen im Gewebe 55fach (Norfloxacin), 61fach (Enoxacin) und 533fach (Ciprofloxacin) über der MHK_{90}.

Schlußfolgerungen

Tierexperimentell erhobene Befunde können nur mit Vorbehalten auf den Menschen übertragen werden. Aufgrund der hohen Gewebekonzentrationen in der Prostata des Hundes und des Menschen sowie des breiten antibakteriellen Spektrums erscheinen die neueren Chinolone vielversprechend in der Behandlung der chronisch bakteriellen Prostatitis.

Literatur

1. **Barry, A. L., R. N. Jones, C. Thornsberry, L. W. Ayers, E. H. Gerlach, H. M. Sommers.** 1984. Antibacterial Activities of Ciprofloxacin, Norfloxacin, Oxolinic Acid, Cinoxacin, and Nalidixic Acid. Antimicrob. Agents Chemother. 25: 633–637.
2. **Bergeron, M. G., M. Thabet, R. Roy, C. Lessard, P. Foucault.** 1985. Norfloxacin Penetration into Human Renal and Prostatic Tissues. Antimicrob. Agents Chemother. 28: 349–350.
3. **Boerema, J. B. J., A. Dalhoff, F. M. Y. Debruyne.** 1985. Ciprofloxacin Distribution in Prostatic Tissue and Fluid Following Oral Administration. Chemotherapy 31: 13–18.
4. **Chin, N.-X., H.-C. Neu.** 1983. In Vitro Activity of Enoxacin, a Quinolone Carboxylic Acid, Compared with those of Norfloxacin, New β-Lactams, Aminoglycosides and Trimethoprim. Antimicrob. Agents Chemother. 24: 754–763.
5. **Fair, W. R., J. J. Cordonnier.** 1978. The pH of Prostatic Fluid: A Reappraisal and Therapeutic Implication. J. Urol. 120: 695–698.
6. **Jacobus, N. V., F. P. Tally, M. Barza.** 1984. Antimicrobial Spectrum of Win 49375. Antimicrob. Agents Chemother. 26: 104–107.
7. **Larsen, E. H., T. C. Gasser, T. Dørflinger, P. O. Madsen.** 1986. The Concentration of Various Quinolone Derivatives in the Human Prostate. In W. Weidner (Ed.) Therapy of Prostatitis, Experimental and Clinical Data. Zuckschwerdt, München, in press.
8. **Madsen, P. O., A. Baumüller, U. Hoyme.** 1978. Experimental Models for Determination of Anti-

microbials in Prostatic Tissue, Interstitial Fluid and Secretion. Scand. J. Infect. Dis. Suppl. 14: 145–150.

9. **Meares, E. M., Jr.** 1980. Prostatitis Syndromes: New Perspectives about Old Woes. J. Urol. 123: 141–147.

10. **Stamey, T. A., E. M. Meares Jr., D. G. Winningham.** 1970. Chronic Bacterial Prostatitis and the Diffusion of Drugs into Prostatic Fluid. J. Urol. 103: 187–194.

11. **Sterling-Winthrop Research Institute.** 1979. A Summary of Laboratory Data for Roxadyl (Brand of Rosoxacin) Injection. Sterling-Winthrop Research Institute, Rensselaer, New York.

12. **Wolfson, J. S., D. C. Hooper.** 1985. The Fluoroquinolones: Structures, Mechanisms of Action and Resistance, and Spectra of Activity In Vitro. Antimicrob. Agents Chemother. 28: 581–586.

ANTIMICROBIAL AGENTS AND CHEMOTHERAPY, May 1987, p. 709–712 Vol. 31, No. 5
0066-4804/87/050709-04$02.00/0

Ciprofloxacin Pharmacokinetics in Patients with Normal and Impaired Renal Function

THOMAS C. GASSER,[1] STEVEN C. EBERT,[2] PEDER H. GRAVERSEN,[1] AND PAUL O. MADSEN[1]*

Urology Section, Surgical Service, William S. Middleton Memorial Veterans Hospital, Madison, Wisconsin 53705,[1] and School of Pharmacy, University of Wisconsin, Madison, Wisconsin 53706[2]

Received 2 September 1986/Accepted 12 February 1987

The pharmacokinetics of ciprofloxacin following single oral doses of 500 and 750 mg in 32 patients with various degrees of renal function impairment were investigated in an open, randomized crossover fashion. Ciprofloxacin was administered after overnight fasting; the washout time between the two doses was 1 week. Serum and urine samples were collected serially between 0 and 24 h and subjected to bioassay and high-performance liquid chromatography. Pharmacokinetic parameters were analyzed, assuming an open two-compartment model with first-order input and elimination. A distinct difference was observed in pharmacokinetic parameters between patients with impaired renal function (creatinine clearance, <50 ml/min per 1.73 m²) and those with normal renal function (creatinine clearance, ≥50 ml/min per 1.73 m²). For the former group, the area under the curve of serum concentration versus time was doubled, the renal clearance of ciprofloxacin was cut to one-fourth, the total and nonrenal ciprofloxacin clearance was reduced by 50%, and the elimination half-life was prolonged by a factor of approximately 1.7. The correlation between renal drug clearance and creatinine clearance was highly significant ($r = 0.890$; $P < 0.001$). On the basis of these findings, it appears that a 50% dose reduction of ciprofloxacin in patients with impaired renal function (creatinine clearance, <50 ml/min per 1.73 m²) may be indicated to achieve concentrations in serum similar to those observed in normal individuals. As the concentration of ciprofloxacin in urine after 24 h remained above the MIC for most urinary pathogens, this drug appears to be of potential benefit for the treatment of urinary tract infections in patients with impaired renal function.

Ciprofloxacin (Bay o 9867) is a new quinolone carboxylic acid derivative with broad antibacterial activity against gram-positive and gram-negative bacteria, including those resistant to aminoglycosides and β-lactam antibiotics (1, 12). Single- and multiple-oral-dose pharmacokinetic studies have shown that ciprofloxacin is rapidly absorbed and penetrates well into tissue (3, 5). Ciprofloxacin is eliminated from serum by renal excretion and by extrarenal routes (11). The purpose of this study was to investigate the pharmacokinetics of ciprofloxacin following single oral doses of 500 and 750 mg in patients with various degrees of renal function.

MATERIALS AND METHODS

Volunteers. Thirty-eight male patients with no known allergies to quinolone derivatives were enrolled in this study after written informed consent was obtained. Six of these subjects were subsequently excluded from analysis from both phases of the study (one vomited shortly after drug administration, one could not be assigned to a group because he had contradictory creatinine clearance [CL_{CR}] values, two had received magnesium hydroxide before drug administration, one received Metamucil, and one ingested food before drug administration). Of the remaining 32 subjects, 4 (2 in each dosing group) were included in analysis in only one phase of the study because they had received magnesium hydroxide on one study day.

The renal function was estimated by CL_{CR} determinations, with two 12-h urinary creatinine collections and two determinations of creatinine in serum prior to ciprofloxacin administration. Patients were initially assigned into four different groups according to their CL_{CR} values: group A, >80 ml/min per 1.73 m² (12 patients); group B, 50 to 79 ml/min per 1.73 m² (5 patients); group C, 20 to 49 ml/min per 1.73 m² (10 patients); and group D, <20 ml/min per 1.73 m² (5 patients). However, during subsequent analysis of these groups, it became obvious that there were no noticeable differences in pharmacokinetic parameters between groups A and B, and between groups C and D. Therefore, patients were reassigned to groups 1 and 2 with CL_{CR} of ≥50 ml/min per 1.73 m² and <50 ml/min per 1.73 m², respectively, for statistical evaluation of pharmacokinetic parameters (Table 1). Most patients had lower-urinary-tract obstruction because of carcinoma of the prostate, hypertrophy of the prostate, or bladder tumors, and some had indwelling urinary catheters.

Study design. This study was an open, randomized crossover trial. Patients received either 500 mg of ciprofloxacin as a single oral dose with at least 7 days of washout time, followed by 750 mg of ciprofloxacin as a single oral dose, or vice versa. The drug was administered with 180 ml of tap water after an overnight fast. Patients were instructed to void before drug administration and to abstain from eating for 4 h after drug administration.

Drug safety was evaluated by measuring vital signs and by questioning the patients about side effects. The following parameters were also measured before and after ciprofloxacin administration: erythrocyte and leukocyte

TABLE 1. Personal data on study subjects

Group (no. of members)	Age range (yr) (median)	Wt range (kg) (median)	CL_{CR} (ml/min per 1.73 m²) (range)
1 (17)	39–74 (60)	64–108 (76)	≥50 (51–157)
2 (15)	48–90 (70)	57–114 (77)	<50 (8–46)

* Corresponding author.

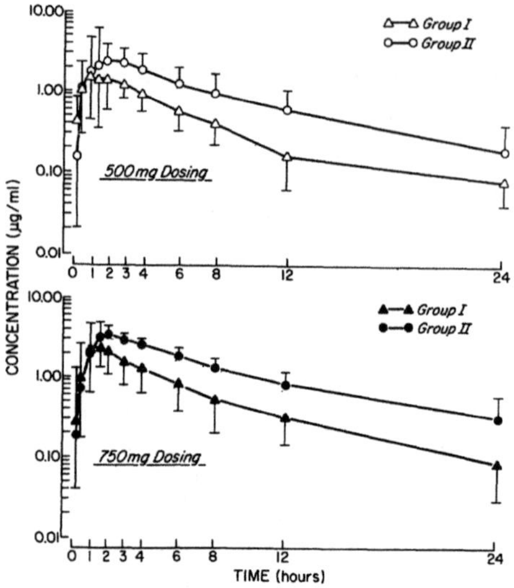

FIG. 1. Ciprofloxacin concentrations in serum after a single oral dose of 500 mg (top) or 750 mg (bottom) (geometric mean and standard deviation).

count, hemoglobin, hematocrit, platelet count, electrolytes, liver enzymes (bilirubin, alkaline phosphatase, serum glutamic oxalacetic transaminase, and serum glutamic pyruvic transaminase), serum creatinine, blood urea nitrogen, uric acid, total protein and albumin, and urinalysis.

Serum samples were drawn before dosing and at 0.25, 0.5, 1.0, 1.5, 2.0, 3.0, 4.0, 6.0, 8.0, 12.0, and 24.0 h after ciprofloxacin administration. Urine was collected before dosing and during the intervals from 0 to 2, 2 to 4, 4 to 8, 8 to 12, and 12 to 24 h thereafter. Urine samples were also taken 24 to 48 h after drug administration in group 2 only. Samples for bioassay were immediately frozen in plastic containers at −20°C; those for high-performance liquid chromatography (HPLC) were frozen at −70°C. All samples were assayed by both bioassay and HPLC.

Microbiological assay. Serum and urine samples were assayed by a plate diffusion method (10), with *Klebsiella pneumoniae* ATCC 10031 (Miles Pharmaceuticals, West Haven, Conn.) as a test organism. The test medium was neomycin assay agar at pH 7.9 (medium 11; Difco Laboratories, Detroit, Mich.). Standards were prepared with pooled normal human antibiotic-free serum for serum samples and a pH 7.0- phosphate buffer for urine. The plates were incubated overnight at 37°C. The standards, controls, and samples were run at least four times. The sensitivity of the assay was 0.01 µg/ml.

HPLC. HPLC serum assay procedures were performed by Miles Pharmaceuticals by a previously described reversed-phase method with fluorescence detection (4). The sensitivity of the assay was 0.008 µg/ml. Urine samples were assayed by a newly developed HPLC method to differentiate between ciprofloxacin and its three metabolites (G. J. Krol, A. J. Noi, and D. Beermann, J. Liq. Chromatogr., in press). Assay results by microbiological and HPLC methods were analyzed for comparability.

Pharmacokinetic analysis. The pharmacokinetic parameters of each subject were individually calculated by nonlinear least-squares regression analysis with a NONLIN program on an IBM-XT personal computer (C. M. Metzler, G. K. Elfring, and A. J. McEwen, Abstr. Biometrics 1984, 2215, p. 562–563).

The pharmacokinetic analysis of the serum values was based on an open, two-compartment model with first-order input and elimination, corresponding to the following equation (6):

$$C_p(t) = Ae^{-\alpha t} + Be^{-\beta t} + Ce^{-k_a t}$$

where $C_p(t)$ (in micrograms per milliliter) is the concentration in serum at time t, A and B (in micrograms per milliliter) are the zero intercepts of the tangents α and β with the y axis, C is $-(A + B)$, α and β (in reciprocal hours) are the slopes of the rapid initial distribution and the slow terminal elimination phases, respectively, and k_a is the absorption rate constant. The secondary parameters, i.e., area under the concentration-time curve from time zero to infinity ($AUC_{0-\infty}$), peak concentration (C_{max}), time at which C_{max} is achieved (T_{max}), distribution and elimination half-lives ($t_{1/2\alpha}$ and $t_{1/2\beta}$, respectively), and volume of the central compartment (V_1) were calculated from the initial parameters (A, B, α, and β) by standard methods (6). The systemic or total drug clearance (CL_{tot}) and the renal drug clearance (CL_R) were calculated from the relationship of dose/$AUC_{0-\infty}$ and $X_u/AUC_{0-\infty}$, respectively, where X_u is the total amount of unchanged drug excreted in the urine. Extrarenal clearance was defined as $C_{NR} = CL_{tot} - CL_R$. The predicted average steady-state concentration in serum was calculated as $AUC_{0-\infty}/T$, where T is the dosage interval.

Statistical analysis. The Wilcoxon rank sum test was used to compare pharmacokinetic parameters between the two groups of patients. The paired t tests was used to test changes in laboratory values.

RESULTS

In both groups 1 and 2, there were excellent correlations between HPLC values and bioassay values for serum (group 1: $r = 0.959$, $y = 0.15 + 0.85x$, $P < 0.001$; and group 2: $r = 0.94$, $y = 0.125 + 0.95x$, $P < 0.001$). Measurement of bias by comparing values from bioassay with those from HPLC revealed a mean difference of only 2.7% for samples in group 1 (310 paired observations) and 2.9% for samples in group 2 (271 paired observations). The correlation of values was not as good for urine ($r = 0.610$, $y = 29 + 0.59x$, $P < 0.001$; mean difference, 19.3%), with bioassay values being higher, probably owing to excretion of biologically active metabolites. These results were consistent with findings of previous studies (9). Therefore, we used bioassay results for serum and HPLC results for urine in our analyses.

Mean concentrations of ciprofloxacin in serum after 500- and 750-mg doses had been given to patients in groups 1 and 2 are shown in Fig. 1. In both groups, the 750-mg dose led to higher levels of ciprofloxacin in serum, higher C_{max}, longer T_{max}, and higher $AUC_{0-\infty}$ than the 500-mg dose (Table 2). Other parameters such as $t_{1/2}$, CL_{tot}, CL_R, and CL_{NR} were dose independent.

Patients in group 2 (those with impaired renal function) had higher dose concentrations in serum than those in group 1 (those with normal or slightly impaired renal function) after both doses. Compared with group 1, group 2 patients also had higher mean values for C_{max} and longer T_{max} (Table 2).

TABLE 2. Pharmacokinetic parameters for ciprofloxacin in patients with normal and impaired renal function[a]

Dose and group (no. of members)	C_{max} (μg/ml)	T_{max} (h)	V_1 (liters)	$t_{1/2\alpha}$ (h)	$t_{1/2\beta}$ (h)	$AUC_{0-\infty}$ (μg · h/ml)	CL_{tot}/F[b] (ml/min)	CL_R/F (ml/min)	CL_{NR}/F (ml/min)
500 mg									
Group 1 (13)	2.2 ± 1.1	1.3 ± 1.0	123.4 ± 46.5	0.65 ± 0.30	4.3 ± 2.5	9.8 ± 4.0	1,002 ± 463	245 ± 101	780 ± 446
Group 2 (14)	2.5 ± 0.8 (NS)[c]	1.8 ± 0.5 ($P < 0.01$)	136.6 ± 11.7 (NS)	0.86 ± 0.61 (NS)	7.1 ± 2.9 ($P < 0.01$)	20.2 ± 9.9 ($P < 0.01$)	527 ± 288 ($P < 0.01$)	64 ± 62 ($P < 0.01$)	462 ± 294 ($P < 0.05$)
750 mg									
Group 1 (13)	2.8 ± 1.5	1.6 ± 0.5	158.0 ± 46.5	0.79 ± 0.35	3.5 ± 1.2	15.6 ± 9.1	1,173 ± 815	272 ± 160	901 ± 699
Group 2 (15)	3.7 ± 0.8 ($P < 0.01$)	2.3 ± 0.8 ($P < 0.01$)	113.8 ± 34.2 (NS)	1.02 ± 0.47 (NS)	6.3 ± 3.2 ($P < 0.01$)	26.8 ± 6.6 ($P < 0.01$)	490 ± 107 ($P < 0.01$)	72 ± 53 ($P < 0.01$)	419 ± 92 ($P < 0.05$)

[a] Results are expressed as the mean ± standard deviation.
[b] F, Bioavailability.
[c] NS, not significant.

The $AUC_{0-\infty}$ was approximately doubled, and $t_{1/2\beta}$ was prolonged by a factor of approximately 1.7. Group 2 patients had statistically smaller CL_{tot}, CL_R, and CL_{NR}. The predicted average concentrations in serum at steady state, assuming a 12-h dosage interval, were as follows: 500-mg dose: 0.82 μg/ml in group 1, 1.68 μg/ml in group 2; 750-mg dose: 1.30 μg/ml in group 1, 2.23 μg/ml in group 2.

The cumulative percentage of ciprofloxacin excreted and unchanged in the urine is shown in Fig. 2. While the percentage of excretion in urine was dose independent, it was only 15% of the dose administered to group 2 patients compared with 26% for group 1 patients. Concentrations in urine after administration of 500 mg of ciprofloxacin are shown in Fig. 3. Renal clearance of ciprofloxacin as a function of endogenous CL_{CR} is shown in Fig. 4. The correlation coefficient ($r = 0.890$) was highly significant ($P < 0.001$).

Ciprofloxacin was well tolerated by nearly all subjects. Four patients in the group given 500 mg and three in the group given 750 mg complained of side effects including headache, dizziness, nausea, vomiting, and diarrhea. Two of the patients experienced severe headache and diarrhea, while the remaining side effects were only of mild intensity, with no differences between groups 1 and 2. No significant changes occurred in the measured laboratory results before and after ciprofloxacin administration.

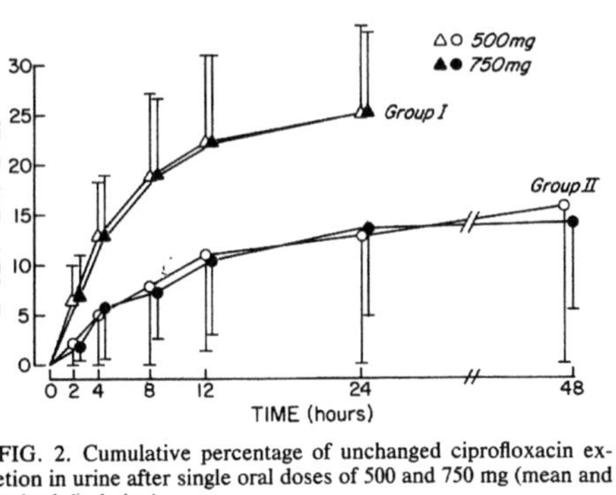

FIG. 2. Cumulative percentage of unchanged ciprofloxacin excretion in urine after single oral doses of 500 and 750 mg (mean and standard deviation).

DISCUSSION

This study demonstrates the relationship between the degree of renal function and ciprofloxacin clearance. Patients with moderate or severely impaired renal function ($CL_{CR} < 50$ ml/min per 1.73 m^2) experienced pharmacokinetic changes with ciprofloxacin administration compared with patients with normal or slightly impaired renal function ($CL_{CR} \geq 50$ ml/min per 1.73 m^2).

Patients with renal function impairment had higher C_{max} and longer T_{max} values, as well as a higher predicted average of steady-state concentrations of ciprofloxacin in serum. Assuming that the bioavailability of ciprofloxacin was the same in both groups, the total ciprofloxacin clearance was greatly reduced in group 2 patients, primarily owing to the lower CL_R. However, CL_{NR} was also significantly reduced in group 2 patients. This may be because the patients in this group were older, often bedridden, and in generally poor physical condition. Reduced CL_R in group 2 patients resulted in a 50% reduction in excretion of unchanged ciprofloxacin in urine. However, the 24-h ciprofloxacin concentration in urine for this group (Fig. 4) was still between 2 and 100 times the MIC for most urinary-tract pathogens, indicating that therapeutic ciprofloxacin levels in urine can be achieved in patients with renal dysfunction and that doses as high as 500 and 750 mg might not be necessary

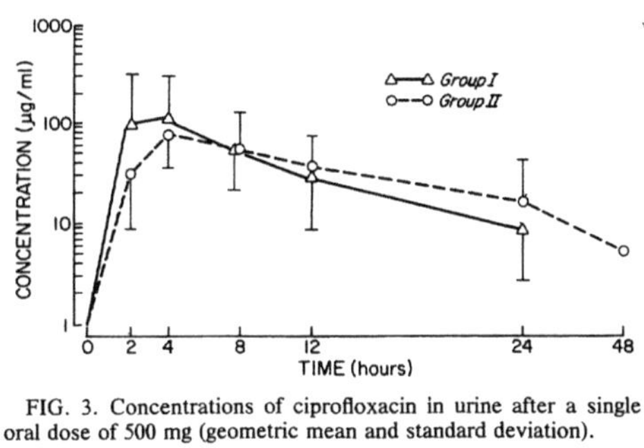

FIG. 3. Concentrations of ciprofloxacin in urine after a single oral dose of 500 mg (geometric mean and standard deviation).

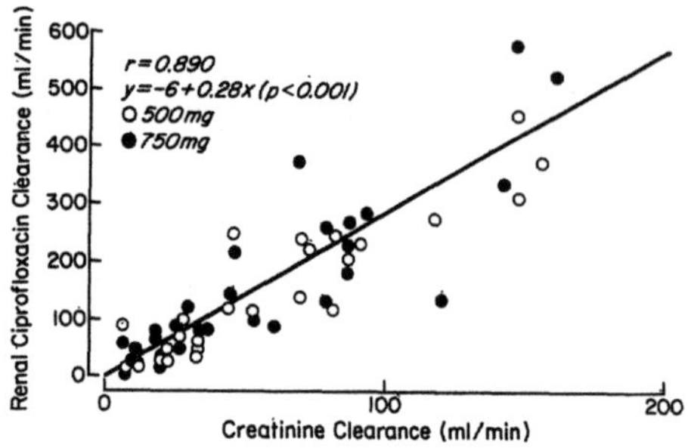

FIG. 4. Correlation between CL_R of ciprofloxacin and endogenous CL_{CR}.

for the treatment of urinary-tract infections in normal individuals.

The absorption of ciprofloxacin did not appear to be influenced by the age of the patients: the C_{max} and T_{max} values were consistent with those from studies of younger patients (11). The extent of absorption as a function of age or renal function was not determined. Other studies have revealed bioavailability values of 60 to 80% (7, 11).

Our study included only male subjects. However, since ciprofloxacin concentrations in serum and urine were sex independent in healthy volunteers in another study (8), we can assume that this would also be true for female patients with impaired renal function.

A study involving the administration of 250 mg of ciprofloxacin to patients with renal failure (CL_{CR}, <20 ml/min per 1.73 m^2) demonstrated alterations in pharmacokinetic parameters similar to those in this study (2). A 50% dose reduction was recommended for these patients. However, since only patients with CL_{CR} of either >60 ml/min per 1.73 m^2 or <20 ml/min per 1.73 m^2 were included in the study, dosage adjustment in patients with CL_{CR} between 20 and 60 ml/min per 1.73 m^2 was not addressed. On the basis of results of our study, the difference of the AUC for serum (and consequently the CL_{tot}) between groups suggests that dose adjustments should be considered for patients with impaired renal function. A reduction in the ciprofloxacin dose by 50% appears indicated for patients with CL_{CR} of <50 ml/min per 1.73 m^2 if concentrations in serum comparable to those in sera of individuals with normal renal function are desired. The high CL_{NR} of cirprofloxacin relative to CL_R, which is consistent with previous studies (11), confirms the importance of extrarenal elimination routes for ciprofloxacin. Therefore, further dose reduction should probably be considered for patients with both impaired renal and impaired hepatic function.

ACKNOWLEDGMENTS

This work was supported in part by the Veterans Administration. We thank Pat Rhodes for her assistance.

LITERATURE CITED

1. **Bauernfeind, A., and C. Petermüller.** 1983. In vitro activity of ciprofloxacin, norfloxacin and nalidixic acid. Eur. J. Clin. Microbiol. 2:111–115.
2. **Boelaert, J., Y. Valcke, M. Schurgers, R. Daneels, M. Rosseneu, M. T. Rosseel, and M. G. Bogaert.** 1985. The pharmacokinetics of ciprofloxacin in patients with impaired renal function. J. Antimicrob. Chemother. 16:87–93.
3. **Crump, B., R. Wise, and J. Dent.** 1983. Pharmacokinetics and tissue penetration of ciprofloxacin. Antimicrob. Agents Chemother. 24:784–786.
4. **Gau, W., H. J. Ploschke, K. Schmidt, and B. Weber.** 1985. Determination of ciprofloxacin (Bay 0 9867) in biological fluids by high-performance liquid chromatography. J. Liq. Chromatogr. 8:485–497.
5. **Gonzalez, M. A., F. Uribe, S. D. Moisen, A. P. Fuster, A. Selen, P. G. Welling, and B. Painter.** 1984. Multiple-dose pharmacokinetics and safety of ciprofloxacin in normal volunteers. Antimicrob. Agents Chemother. 26:741–744.
6. **Greenblatt, D. J., and J. Koch-Weser.** 1975. Drug therapy. Clinical pharmacokinetics (part 1). N. Engl. J. Med. 293:702–705.
7. **Höffken, G., H. Lode, C. Prinzing, K. Borner, and P. Koeppe.** 1985. Pharmacokinetics of ciprofloxacin after oral and parenteral administration. Antimicrob. Agents Chemother. 27:375–379.
8. **Höffler, D., A. Dalhoff, W. Gau, D. Beermann, and A. Michl.** 1984. Dose- and sex-independent disposition of ciprofloxacin. Eur. J. Clin. Microbiol. 3:363–366.
9. **Joos, B., B. Ledergerber, M. Flepp, J.-D. Bettex, R. Lüthy, and W. Siegenthaler.** 1985. Comparison of high-pressure liquid chromatography and bioassay for determination of ciprofloxacin in serum and urine. Antimicrob. Agents Chemother. 27:353–356.
10. **Washington, J. A., II, and V. L. Sutter.** 1980. Dilution susceptibility test: agar and macro-broth dilution procedures, p. 453–458. *In* E. H. Lennette, A. Balows, W. J. Hausler, Jr., and J. P. Truant (ed.), Manual of clinical microbiology, 3rd ed. American Society for Microbiology, Washington, D.C.
11. **Wingender, W., K.-H. Graefe, W. Gau, D. Förster, D. Beermann, and P. Schacht.** 1984. Pharmacokinetics of ciprofloxacin after oral and intravenous administration in healthy volunteers. Eur. J. Clin. Microbiol. 3:355–359.
12. **Wise, R., J. M. Andrews, and L. J. Edwards.** 1983. In vitro activity of Bay 09867, a new quinoline derivative, compared with those of other antimicrobial agents. Antimicrob. Agents Chemother. 23:559–564.

Treatment of Complicated Urinary Tract Infections with Ciprofloxacin

THOMAS C. GASSER, M.D.
PEDER H. GRAVERSEN, M.D.
PAUL O. MADSEN, M.D.
Madison, Wisconsin

The safety and efficacy of three different dosage regimens of ciprofloxacin (250, 500, and 750 mg orally every 12 hours for seven days) were compared in a prospective, controlled, randomized, double-blind study. Enrolled were 161 patients (110 who were evaluable for efficacy) with complicated urinary tract infection defined as a bacterial count of at least 10^5 colony-forming units/ml of urine in the presence of structural or functional abnormality of the urinary tract. Cure rates five to nine days after treatment were 84 percent, 87 percent, and 86 percent in the 250-, 500-, and 750-mg dosage groups, respectively, with no significant difference between groups. This suggests that 250 mg of ciprofloxacin twice daily is sufficient for the treatment of urinary tract infection. All three dosage regimens were well tolerated.

Ciprofloxacin is a new quinolone with a broad antibacterial spectrum against gram-positive and gram-negative organisms, including Enterobacteriaceae and strains of Pseudomonas aeruginosa [1]. After oral administration, the drug rapidly achieves high levels in the urine [2], and it is therefore expected to be effective as a treatment for urinary tract infection. To investigate the safety and efficacy of ciprofloxacin, a comparison of three oral dosage regimens was carried out.

PATIENTS AND METHODS

Five women and 156 men (161 patients) with complicated urinary tract infections were enrolled in a prospective, controlled, randomized, double-blind study. All 161 were evaluable for safety; 110 were evaluable for efficacy. Fifty-one patients were excluded for the following reasons: 20 had negative urine culture results before treatment; 22 had no urine specimens cultured during or after treatment; and nine had taken the medication incorrectly. Complicated urinary tract infection was defined as a bacterial count of at least 10^5 colony-forming units (cfu)/ml of urine in the presence of structural or functional abnormality of the urinary tract, accompanied by typical signs and symptoms of infection. Patients were randomly assigned to receive treatment with either 250, 500, or 750 mg of oral ciprofloxacin every 12 hours for seven days. Urine specimens were cultured before, during, and five to nine days after therapy. The bacteriologic response five to nine days after treatment was defined as follows: cure, less than 10^5 cfu/ml of urine of the same organism; persistence, at least 10^5 cfu/ml of the same organism; reinfection, at least 10^5 cfu/ml of a new organism; and superinfection, at least 10^5 cfu/ml with a new organism in addition to the original one. For the safety evaluation, the incidence of side effects was recorded, and laboratory tests of hematologic and blood chemistry parameters (including kidney function parameters and liver enzymes) and urinalysis were performed before, during, and 48 hours after treatment.

From the William S. Middleton Memorial Veterans Hospital and University of Wisconsin Medical School, Madison, Wisconsin. This work was supported in part by funds from the United States Veterans Administration. Requests for reprints should be addressed to Dr. Paul O. Madsen, Urology Section, William S. Middleton Memorial Veterans Hospital, 2500 Overlook Terrace, Madison, Wisconsin 53705.

The three treatment groups were comparable in age, weight, and urologic diagnosis of the patients (**Table I**). The most common causative organism was Escherichia coli (35 strains). This was followed by Streptococcus species (28), Pseudomonas species (22), Staphylococcus species (18), Enterobacter cloacae (six), Klebsiella pneumoniae (five), Proteus mirabilis (four), and others (Candida albicans, Alcaligenes odorans, Citrobacter freundii, Gardnerella vaginalis) (five). Eleven patients had more than one type of organism. There was no difference between the treatment groups.

RESULTS

The bacteriologic results are summarized in **Table II**. There was no significant difference in cure rates between the treatment groups. The 15 persistent infections comprised five P. aeruginosa, five Streptococcus faecalis, two C. albicans, one P. mirabilis, one E. cloacae, and one A. odorans. One patient with E. coli became reinfected with S. faecalis. One patient with P. aeruginosa became superinfected with S. faecalis, and one patient with S. faecalis was superinfected with Serratia marcescens.

Ciprofloxacin was well tolerated. Values of laboratory parameters were not altered. Adverse reactions considered probably or possibly due to treatment with ciprofloxacin occurred in 18 of the 161 patients (11 percent): five gastrointestinal, six neurologic, six gastrointestinal and neurologic, and one skin rash. There were no differences between groups. Only one patient, whose previously present gastrointestinal symptoms were worsened by the drug, required discontinuation of therapy.

In this study, ciprofloxacin has been shown to be highly effective in the treatment of complicated urinary tract infection. Cure rates of 85 percent five to nine days after completion of therapy are considered excellent in our patient population. Similar cure rates (82 percent) were found in an earlier open study of 28 patients with complicated urinary tract infections [3]. Moreover, cure rates of 89 percent have been found in patients with urinary tract infections caused by P. aeruginosa [4], a notoriously difficult pathogen to treat.

There was no difference in bacteriologic results between the treatment groups. This is not surprising, considering the high levels of ciprofloxacin in the urine and the low minimal inhibitory concentration against most urinary pathogens. It appears, therefore, that 250 mg of oral ciprofloxacin twice daily for seven days is sufficient for the treatment of complicated urinary tract infection. In addition, ciprofloxacin seems to be a safe drug, as all three dosage regimens were well tolerated.

TABLE I Patient Characteristics and Distribution of Diagnoses

	Dose (mg)		
	250 (n = 38)	500 (n = 34)	750 (n = 38)
Age (years, mean ± SD)	65.2 ± 11.2	68.8 ± 11.1	65.9 ± 10.4
Weight (kg, mean ± SD)	81.7 ± 17.7	80.5 ± 17.4	77.1 ± 17.8
Diagnosis (number)*			
Benign prostatic hyperplasia	21	19	17
Carcinoma of prostate	5	5	7
Carcinoma of bladder	7	1	4
Urethral stricture	5	6	7
Bladder neck contracture	2	0	2
Neurogenic bladder	1	3	3
Others†	3	7	5

*Fifteen patients had more than one diagnosis.
†Includes calculi, phimosis, carcinoma of penis, epididymitis, and interstitial cystitis (non-infectious bladder disease).

REFERENCES

1. Barry AL, Jones RN, Thornsberry C, Ayers LW, Gerlach EH, Sommers HM: Antibacterial activities of ciprofloxacin, norfloxacin, oxolinic acid, cinoxacin, and nalidixic acid. Antimicrob Agents Chemother 1984; 25: 633–637.
2. Höffken G, Lode H, Prinzing C, Borner K, Koeppe P: Pharmacokinetics of ciprofloxacin after oral and parenteral administration. Antimicrob Agents Chemother 1985; 27: 375–379.
3. Boerema J, Boll B, Muytjens H, Branolte J: Efficacy and safety of ciprofloxacin (Bay o 9867) in the treatment of patients with complicated urinary tract infection. J Antimicrob Chemother 1985; 16: 211–217.
4. Scully BE, Neu HC, Parry MF, Mandell W: Oral ciprofloxacin therapy of infections due to Pseudomonas aeruginosa. Lancet 1986; I: 819–822.

TABLE II Bacteriologic Results

	Number of Patients (percent)					
	Dose (mg)					
	250		500		750	
Response*	Day 3	Follow-Up†	Day 3	Follow-Up†	Day 3	Follow-Up†
Cure	42 (98)	36 (84)	36 (97)	32 (87)	41 (95)	37 (86)
Persistence	1	6	1	4	2	5
Reinfection	0	1	0	0	0	0
Superinfection	0	0	0	1	0	1

*There was no statistical difference between groups (chi-square test).
†Follow-up was five to nine days after treatment.

Reprinted from the April issue of **The American Journal of Medicine,** A Yorke Medical Journal. Published by The Cahners Publishing Company, A Division of Reed Publishing USA, 275 Washington St., Newton, MA 02158-1630.

Antimicrobial Prophylaxis in Urology: Timing, Dosing, and Duration Studies with special reference to High-risk conditions

T. C. Gasser, P. O. Madsen

Summary: A study in guinea pigs was performed to investigate the importance of timing, dosage, and duration of antimicrobial prophylaxis in urologic surgery. To simulate high-risk conditions, in one group a foreign body was implanted subcutaneously. The prostate and one kidney were cauterized and bacteremia was induced by intravenous injection of Escherichia coli solution. Various ciprofloxacin regimen were tested.

The results indicate that antimicrobial prophylaxis is beneficial only if administered before or shortly after surgery. Full therapeutic dosage may not be necessary for prophylactic efficacy. Single dose prophylaxis was as effective as multiple doses. Foreign body infection could be prevented by single-dose prophylaxis.

Introduction

Antimicrobial prophylaxis to prevent infectious complications has been used in surgery for many decades. Over 30 years ago, Burke (1), using cutaneous inoculation with Staphylococcus aureus in guinea pigs, found antimicrobial prophylaxis was effective only during a short decisive period, i.e., from the time the bacteria entered the body until 3 h later. Burke's data have been directly transformed into clinical use and are still applied today.

Antimicrobial prophylaxis is widely used – and possibly misused (2). Increasing numbers of high-risk patients (implantation of foreign bodies, such as joint replacements, pace makers) require urologic surgery. Many new, highly potent antimicrobials such as quinolones have been developed. However, surprisingly few studies have been published regarding basic questions such as timing, duration, and dosing of antimicrobials and their benefits in high-risk patients.

Materials and Methods

Animals: White Hartley guinea pigs (Charmany Farms, Madison, Wisconsin, USA) with a mean weight of 499 g ± 74 were used. The animals were anesthetized with ketamine hydrochloride (60 mg/100 g body weight) and xylazine (6 mg/100 g body weight) intramuscularly. In addition, the skin was anesthetized subcutaneously with a 1 % lidocaine injection. After shaving, the skin was prepared with merthiolate (Eli Lilly, Indianapolis, Indiana, USA).

A lower midline laparotomy was performed. The bladder was punctured with a 25-gauge needle and urine was aspirated for bacterial culture to rule out pre-existing urinary tract infection. To mimic surgery involving electrocautery, the prostate and the left kidney were cauterized. For this, the bladder was opened at its dome, and the prostatic urethra was cauterized with a small electrode for 3 s. The left kidney was exposed and cauterized similarly for 3 s to produce a 4 x 4-mm lesion. The lower vena cava was then exposed for repeat blood aspiration and injection of the antimicrobial or bacterial solution.

Study groups of four to eight animals were used. The animals were sacrificed 24 h after the study with the exception of the foreign body studies, where the animals were sacrificed after 48 h. The liver, spleen, left and right kidney, bladder, and prostate were removed under sterile conditions and examined for bacterial counts. If not stated otherwise, ciprofloxacin (Ciproxin, Bayer) was given at a dose of 5.7 mg/kg.

Bacteremia studies: The bacterial solution was injected into the inferior vena cava. Blood was aspirated before and every 10 min after injection for 1 h and examined for viable bacteria. One group of seven animals received no antimicrobial prophylaxis and served as control group. Another group of seven animals received a single dose of ciprofloxacin 15 min before the bacterial challenge.

Timing studies: Ciprofloxacin was given to four groups of animals: 1) 15 min before (six animals), 2) together with (six animals), 3) 15 min after (seven animals) and 4) 3 hours after (six animals) the bacterial solution .

Dosing studies: To investigate if a smaller dose would be sufficient for the purpose of prophylaxis, ciprofloxacin was injected 15 min before the bacterial solution in three groups of animals at doses of 1) 5.7 mg/kg (full dose) (six animals), 2) 1.4 mg/kg (1/4 dose) (seven animals), and 3) 0.7 mg/kg(1/8 dose) (seven animals).

Duration studies: Ciprofloxacin prophylaxis was given as a single dose before (seven animals) or as three doses before, 3 h, and 6 h after the bacterial challenge (six animals). In addition, one group was treated with a single dose of 5.7 mg/kg fleroxacin (Quinodis, Hoffmann-La Roche) (six animals).

Foreign body studies: In 16 animals two cylindrical plastic chambers (3 x 1 cm, Ciba-Geigy, Basel, Switzerland) were implanted subcutaneously to serve as foreign bodies (3). As each animal carried two chambers, groups of only four animals each were used. The chambers were perforated to allow for repeat aspiration of chamber fluid. After approximately 3 weeks, when the chambers had healed in completely, the animals were injected with the bacterial solution intravenously, and the chambers were punctured at 0, 1, 3, 6, 24, and 48 h. The aspirate was cultured for viable counts. One group of four animals received no antimicrobials. One group of four received ciprofloxacin 15 min before the bacterial challenge. Another two groups of four animals received ciprofloxacin three times and fleroxacin once, respectively. At sacrifice, the chambers were removed and placed in Mueller-Hinton broth for overnight culture.

Preparation of bacterial solution: Escherichia coli ATCC 25922, a commercially available standard strain, was grown overnight in Mueller-Hinton broth (BBL Microbiology Systems, Cockeysville, Massachusetts, USA) and 0.05 ml were diluted in 5 ml normal saline. One-tenth of a milliliter of this solution was injected intravenously, giving a mean inoculum of 2.7×10^5 colony-forming units per millilitre (CFU/ml).

Bacterial counts: For the bacteremia studies, 0.2 ml of blood was drawn. In the control group half of this amount (0.1 ml) was directly streaked out on MacConkey agar (Difco Laboratories, Detroit, Michigan, USA). After incubation overnight at 37 °C, the colonies were counted under a scanning microscope. Only bright red colonies were accepted as Escherichia coli. By multiplying the actual number by 10, the CFU/ml blood were calculated (limit of detection: 10 CFU/ml). To detect low bacteremia, the remaining 0.1 ml of blood was placed overnight in the Mueller-Hinton broth and examined for bacterial growth the next day. In the prophylaxis group the blood was first passed through a bacterial filter (diameter 0.45 µm pore size, Millipore Corp. Milford, Massachusetts, USA) (4). No lyzing solution was used. The filter was rinsed with sterile saline to remove the antimicrobial and then directly placed on agar and grown overnight. The colonies were counted the following day.

To express the bacterial counts in various organs, the organs were placed in preweighed plastic containers containing 2 ml sterile saline, and the weight of the tissue was determined. The tissue was homogenized in a Polytron homogenizer (Kinematica, Lucerne, Switzerland). Serial dilutions of 1:5 were made of the homogenate and 0.01 ml of each dilution was streaked out on MacConkey agar. The plates were incubated overnight at 37 °C, and the number of CFU were counted using a scanning microscope.

Statistics: Fisher's exact test was used for statistical evaluation. A p value of less than 0.05 was considered significant.

Results

The inoculum of 2.7×10^5 CFU/ml caused infections in all organs examined of all animals (Table 1). When 10^4 and 10^3 CFU/ml were used, only approximately 50 % and 20 %, respectively, of the organs became infected. The cauterized left kidney became more often infected than the right one.

After intravenous injection of 2.7×10^5 CFU/ml the bacteremia reached 1.5×10^3 CFU/ml at 10 min and rapidly dropped to numbers below 50 CFU/ml at 60 min (Fig. 1). However, after previous ciprofloxacin injection, no bacteria could be detected in the blood.

Timing study: Figure 2 shows that, with ciprofloxacin and fleroxacin, the infection rate could be reduced significantly. The effect was most pronounced in liver, spleen, and prostate. Prophylaxis was less effective in the bladder and in the cauterized kidney. However, prophylactic efficacy was noted only if ciprofloxacin was given shortly before or after the bacterial challenge. When administered 3 h after induction of bacteremia, infection could not be prevented reliably (no significant difference to controls).

Dosing study: With only one-fourth of the recommended dose a significant reduction of infection was noted in most organs, with the exception of the bladder (Fig. 3). The rate of infection did not significantly differ from the ones found with full ciprofloxacin dose. However, 1/8 of the full dose was not effective in reducing infection (no significant difference to controls).

Table 1. Duration study: Percentage of infected organs after intravenous injection of Escherichia coli

Tissue	Control	Ciprofloxacin	Ciprofloxacin	Fleroxacin
Doses	none	1 time	3 times	1 time
n =	7	7	6	6
Liver	100	0	0	0
Spleen	100	14	0	33
Right kidney	100	29	33	0
Left kidney	100	29	50	50
Bladder	100	0	50	50
Prostate	100	14	16	33

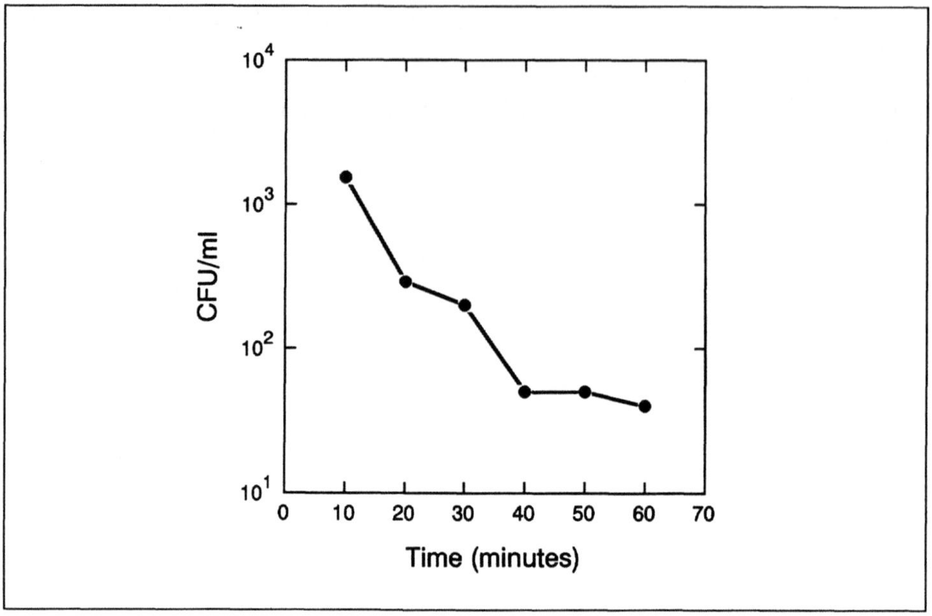

Fig. 1. Bacteremia after intravenous injection of Escherichia coli (median). CFU/ml = colony forming units per milliliter blood.

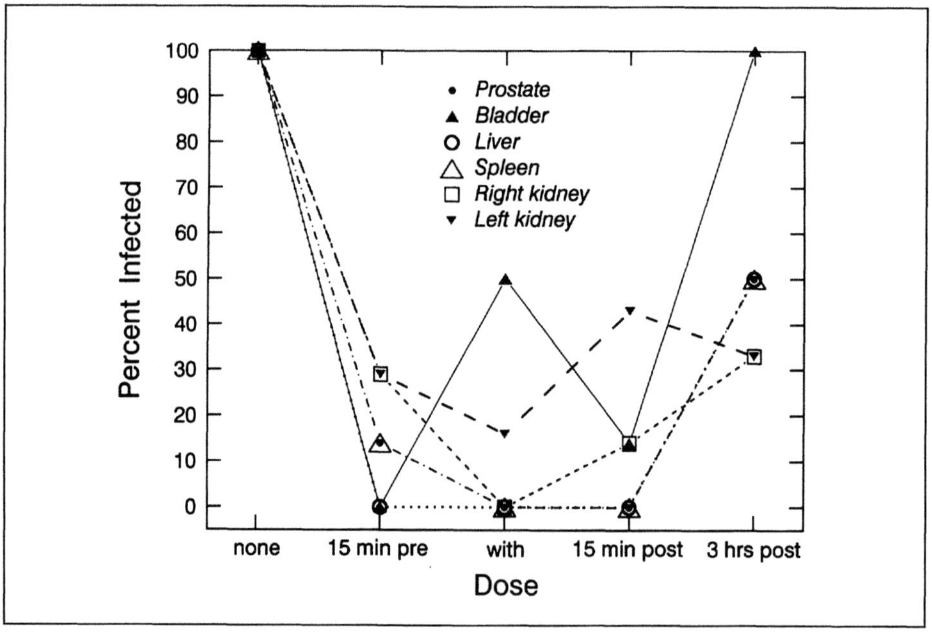

Fig. 2. Timing study. Ciprofloxacin injection 15 min before (pre), simultaneously (with), 15 min and 3 h after (post) the injection of Escherichia coli.

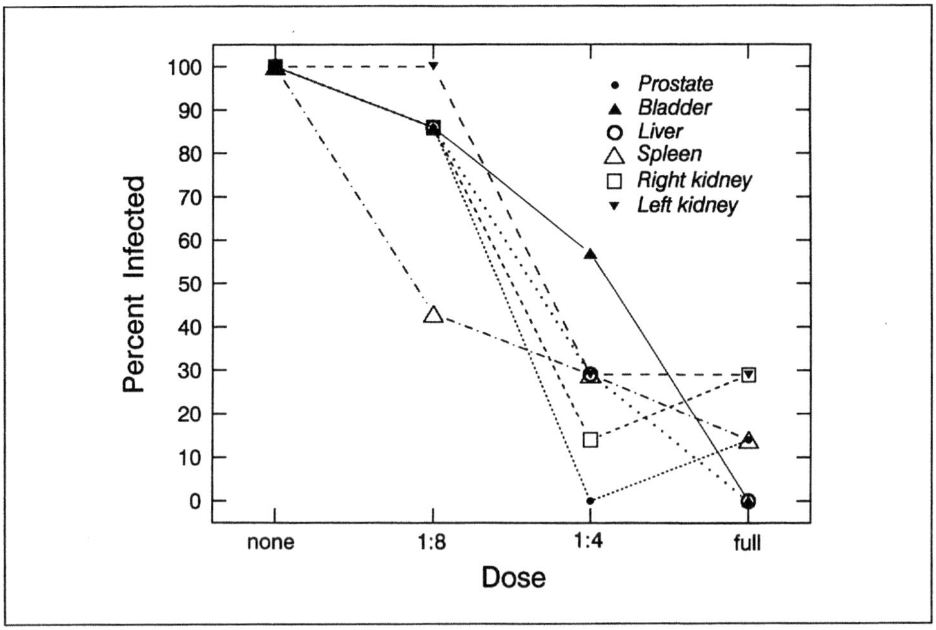

Fig. 3. Dosing study. Ciprofloxacin injection of 1/8, 1/4 and full dose 15-min before injection of Escherichia coli.

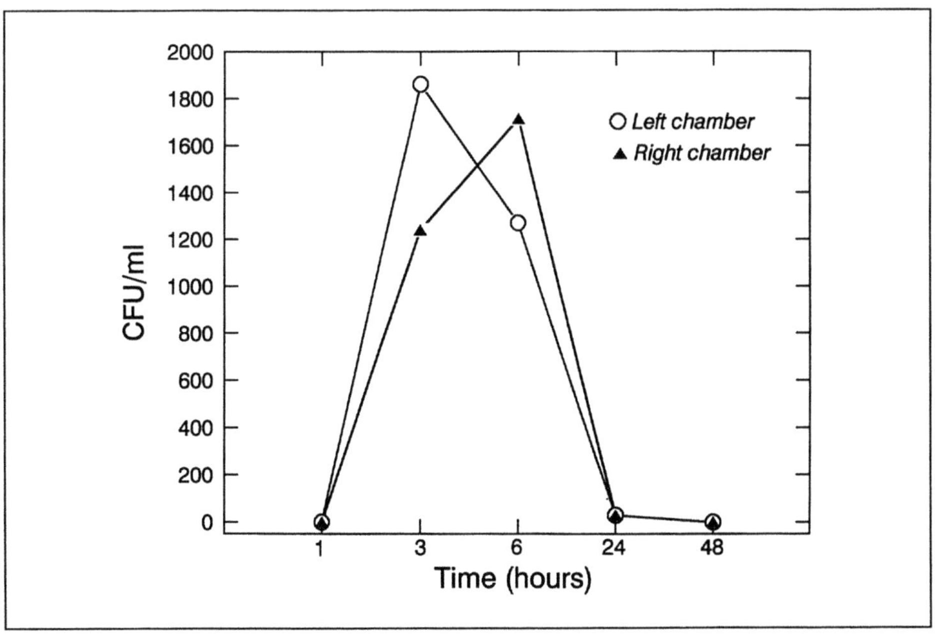

Fig. 4. Foreign body studies. Aspirates of chamber fluid 0, 1, 3, 6, 24, and 48 h after intravenous injection of Escherichia coli (median). CFU/ml = colony forming units per milliliter aspirate.

Duration study: The reduction of infection achieved by a single dose of ciprofloxacin could not be further enhanced by multiple administration. Fleroxacin and ciprofloxacin were equally effective (Table 1).

Foreign body studies: The animals tolerated the implanted chambers well. None of the chambers was infected at the beginning of the experiments. After the intravenous injection of the bacterial solution the chambers did not become infected until 3 h later at which time all the chambers were infected (Fig. 4). The maximal colony count was noted after 6 h. Surprisingly, after 48 h the chamber aspirates and the chambers itself were sterile. Chamber infection could completely be prevented by three doses of ciprofloxacin as no chamber was infected. A single dose of ciprofloxacin or fleroxacin led to sterile chambers in all animals.

Discussion

Over 30 years ago, Burke (1) established the important relation between the timing of an antimicrobial and its prophylactic efficacy. The then used antimicrobials penicillin G potassium, chloramphenicol, erythromycin, and achromycin could prevent infection only if administered during a short decisive period – between the entrance of the bacteria and no later than 3 h thereafter. However, Burke's experiments do not directly relate to urologic surgery for two reasons. First, he used gram – positive organisms rarely encountered in urologic surgery. Second, he performed the prophylactic studies on skin incisions, which is also not applicable to urologic surgery. Possibly for these reasons, Nielsen and Madsen (5) could not confirm the existence of this limited time period, as the antimicrobial used in their study, the cephalosporin cefotaxime, was effective in preventing infections up to 6 h after the bacterial challenge. In their study, the type of infecting organism and infected organ appeared to be of greater importance.

Antimicrobial prophylaxis is used universally in almost every surgical field (2,6). While the benefit of some kind of antimicrobial prophylaxis has been established for many surgical specialties (i.e., orthopedic, vascular, colonic surgery) much controversy remains in urology (7). Moreover, despite the wide use of antimicrobial prophylaxis and the increase of high – risk patients (e.g., patients with prostheses, etc.) surprisingly little experimental research has been published, addressing such important questions as dosing and length of administration of antimicrobials in high-risk conditions.

In this study, we attempted to simulate clinical conditions often encountered in urologic practice. Surgical trauma involving electrocautery (as in transurethral resection) was produced by cauterizing the prostate and the left kidney.

Bacteremia often originates from the urinary tract (7). Bacteremia occurs in up to 60 % of the patients with preoperative bacteriuria undergoing transurethral resection of the prostate (8). In the case of preoperative sterile urine, up to 36 % of the blood cultures are positive (9). As bacteremia poses the real threat to the patient, we induced bacteremia by intravenous injection of a bacterial suspension. The plastic chambers were implanted to mimic a prosthetic device frequently found in older patients.

This guinea – pig study confirms Burke's findings for newer, more potent antimicrobials, like the quinolones, since infection could be prevented reliably. It appears, however, that the decisive period is even shorter than the presently accepted 3 h, supporting the administration of the antimicrobial at the time of induction of anesthesia.

Interestingly, to achieve protection against infection, one- fourth of the recommended therapeutic dose for ciprofloxacin may be sufficient. This may be due to the very low minimal inhibitory concentration of ciprofloxacin against most pathogens encountered in urologic surgery (10). With estimated yearly overall expenses of US$ 15 billion for antimicrobials worldwide (2), administration of a lower antimicrobial single dose for prophylactic purposes would result in considerable cost reduction.

The optimal length of antimicrobial prophylaxis is still debated. In an experimental study, single dose amoxicillin – gentamicin prophylaxis was less effective than multiple doses in preventing streptococcal endocarditis (11). Also, in urology some authors still recommend prophylaxis to be extended for several days, while others stress the single dose regimen (12, 13). This study supports the current trend of using a single dose of an antimicrobial against postoperative infection. Longer administration of the antimicrobial did not yield better results than a single dose. Fleroxacin and ciprofloxacin were equally effective in preventing infection. The half-life of fleroxacin in guinea pigs is similar to ciprofloxacin (1.8 h and 1.5 h, respectively) (14). In humans, however, the half-life of fleroxacin is considerably longer than of ciprofloxacin (11.2 and 3.3 h, respectively) (15). Therefore, from a theoretical standpoint the long half-life of fleroxacin and its excellent tissue penetration would make it an ideal drug for prophylactic purposes, especially for longer operations (16).

Foreign bodies are particularly prone to becoming infected since they represent a locus minoris resistentiae (3, 17). Besides bacterial contamination at the time of insertion the foreign body may become infected hematogenously. We found that intravenously injected bacteria could be recovered from the subcutaneous chambers after 3 h and reached a maximum count after 6 h. However, after 48 h the chamber fluid as well as the chambers itself were sterile, suggesting that the inoculum of 2.7×10^5 CFU/ml was not high enough to establish infection. Zimmerli et al. found that with an inoculum as high as 5×10^8 CFU/ml 82 % of the cages became permanently infected (3). This indicates that extravascular foreign bodies are at risk for hematogenous infection, however, only when exposed to high numbers of bacteria. The incidence of bacteremia during and after transurethral resection of the prostate has been reported as high as 60 % (8). However, the actual bacterial density occurring during a bacteremia is not known. It has been estimated that bacterial concentrations of $10^2 - 10^3$ CFU/ml are frequently encountered in human bacteremia (3). Therefore, the risk of hematogenous infection of an extravascular foreign body appears to be remote and can be practically eliminated by a single dose of ciprofloxacin or fleroxacin.

In conclusion, the necessity to administer the antimicrobial before surgery is confirmed. A single dose of ciprofloxacin or fleroxacin appears to be as effective as multiple doses. Full therapeutic dose may not be necessary for prophylactic efficacy. Foreign bodies are probably infected hematogenously in less than 3 h after the bacterial challenge, but infection can be prevented by single – dose prophylaxis.

Acknowledgment:

We thank Dr. W. Zimmerli for constructive comments, and Pat Rhodes and Jane Knes for excellent technical assistance.
Fleroxacin was provided by Hoffman-La Roche, Inc. Nutley, New Jersey, USA.
This study was supported in part by the Department of Veterans Affairs, USA.

References

1. Burke JF (1961) The effective period of preventive antibiotic action in experimental incisions and dermal lesions. Surgery 50: 161-168
2. Kunin CM, Johansen KS, Worning AM, Daschner FD (1990) Report of a symposium on use and abuse of antibiotics worldwide. Rev Infect Dis 12: 12-19
3. Zimmerli W, Zak O, Vosbeck K. (1985) Experimental hematogenous infection of subcutanously implanted foreign bodies. Scand J Infect Dis 17: 303-310
4. Sullivan NM, Sutter VL, Finegold SM (1975) Practical aerobic membrane filtration blood culture technique: Development of procedure. J Clin Microbiol 1: 30-36
5. Nielsen OS, Madsen PO (1982) Importance and timing of prophylactic antibiotics in urology with a special reference to growth and kill rates of E. coli in genitourinary organs. J Urol 123: 608-614
6. Kaiser AB (1986) Antimicrobial prophylaxis in surgery. N Engl J Med 315: 1129-1138
7. Larsen EH, Gasser TC, Madsen PO (1986) Antimicrobial prophylaxis in urologic surgery. Urol Clin N Am 13: 591-604
8. Murphy DM, Stassen L, Carr ME, Gillespie WA, Cafferkey MT, Falkiner FR (1984) Bactaeremia during prostatectomy and other transurethral operations: influence of timing of antibiotic administration. J Clin Pathol 37: 673-676
9. Robinson MRG, Arudpragasam ST, Sahgal SM, Cross RJ, Akdas A, Fittal B, Sibbald R (1982) Bactaeremia resulting from prostatic surgery: the source of bacteria. Br J Urol 54: 542-546
10. Nielsen KT, Madsen PO (1989) Quinolones in Urology. Urol Res 17: 117-124
11. Malinverni R, Francioli PB, Glauser MP (1987) Comparison of single and multiple doses of prophylactic antibiotics in experimental streptococcus endocarditis. Circulation 76: 376-382
12. Hargreave TB, Gould JC, Kinninmonth AWG, Jeffrey RR, Varma JS, Macintyre CCA, Elton RA, Chisholm GD (1984) A randomized trial of 48 hours of prophylactic cefotaxime versus single dose in transurethral prostatic surgery. J Antimicrob Chemother 14 (suppl B): 263-269
13. Grabe M, Forsgren A, Björk T, Hellsten S (1987) Controlled trial of a short and a prolonged course with ciprofloxacin in patients undergoing transurethral prostatic surgery. Eur J Clin Microbiol 6: 11-17
14. Widmer AF, Wiestner A, Frei R, Zimmerli W (1991) Killing of nongrowing and adherent Escherichia coli determines drug efficacy in device-related infections. Antimicrob Agents Chemother 35: 741-746
15. Hooper DC, Wolfson JS (1991) Fluoroquinolone antimicrobial agents. N Engl J Med 324: 384-394
16. Gasser TC, Graversen PH, Madsen PO (1987) Fleroxacin (Ro 23-6240) distribution in canine prostatic tissue and fluids. Antimicrob Agents Chemother 31: 1010-1013
17. Nickel JC, Heaton J, Morales A, Costerton JW (1986) Bacterial biofilm in persistent penile prosthesis-associated infection. J Urol 135: 586-588

Authors' addresses:

Thomas C. Gasser, M.D.
Urologic Clinics
University Hospital
4031 Basel
Switzerland

Paul O. Madsen, M.D., Ph.D.
Professor of Urology
VA Hospital
2500 Overlook Terrace
Madison, Wisconsin 53705
USA

GPSR Compliance

The European Union's (EU) General Product Safety Regulation (GPSR) is a set of rules that requires consumer products to be safe and our obligations to ensure this.

If you have any concerns about our products, you can contact us on ProductSafety@springernature.com

In case Publisher is established outside the EU, the EU authorized representative is:

Springer Nature Customer Service Center GmbH
Europaplatz 3
69115 Heidelberg, Germany

Batch number: 10577969

Printed by Printforce, the Netherlands